THE META-CENTER'S

HERBAL APOTHECARY

BY TONY VORTEX

First Edition
ISBN 978-1-949432-12-1

Published by:

Inner Alchemy's Publishing (Inner Alchemy's)

332 S. Michigan Ave.
Ste 121-C141
Chicago, IL 60604-4434

info@inneralchemys.com www.inneralchemys.com

Printed in the United States of America

HEALTHCARE DISCLAIMER

CONTENTS

HONEYS

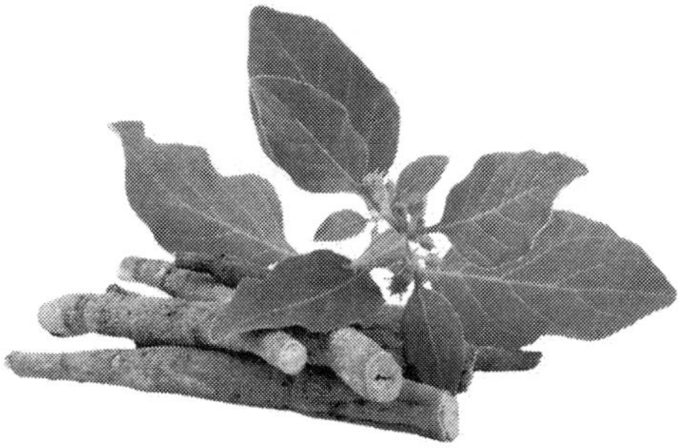

ASHWAGANDHA

(WITHANIA SOMNIFERA)

commonly known as Indian ginseng or winter cherry, is a revered herb in traditional Indian medicine, Ayurveda.

1. DESCRIPTION: Ashwagandha is a small, woody shrub with elliptical green leaves, small, greenish-yellow flowers, and red-orange berries enclosed in papery husks. It typically grows about 30-75 cm in height. Its roots, which are the most utilized part, are stout and long, exuding a characteristic earthy aroma.

2. LOCATION: It is native to India, the Middle East, and parts of Africa. Due to its adaptogenic properties, it is also cultivated in more temperate climates including regions of the United States.

3. GROWING CONDITIONS: Ashwagandha thrives in dry, stony soil with minimal water and full sun exposure. It is drought-tolerant and grows well in arid regions. The plant prefers hot, sunny locations and is relatively resistant to pests.

4. TRADITIONAL USES: Traditionally, Ashwagandha has been used to rejuvenate and restore bodily functions. It is considered a tonic and adaptogen, employed to help the body resist physiological and psychological stress. The roots are used to make powders, teas, and extracts, often used to enhance energy, improve concentration, and increase stamina.

5. SCIENTIFIC BENEFITS: Research on Ashwagandha has shown several potential health benefits, including anti-inflammatory and antioxidant properties, reduction in cortisol levels, improvement in brain function, and relief from anxiety and depression. Studies suggest it may also enhance muscle strength and recovery.

6. METAPHYSICAL USES: In the realm of esoteric and metaphysical practices, Ashwagandha is used for grounding, bringing energy to the physical body, and stabilizing mood. It is believed to harmonize mind, body, and spirit, and is used in rituals to enhance focus and meditation.

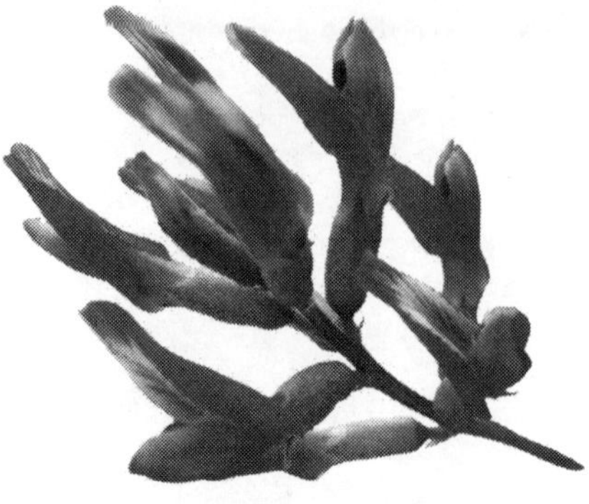

ASTRAGALUS

(ASTRAGALUS MEMBRANACEUS)

also known as milkvetch or huáng qí in Traditional Chinese Medicine, is a perennial plant native to the northern and eastern parts of China as well as Mongolia and Korea.

1. DESCRIPTION: Astragalus is characterized by its long, thin stems, which can grow up to 36 inches tall. The plant produces small, pale-yellow flowers that resemble those of a pea plant, as it belongs to the legume family. Its root, which can grow quite deep into the soil, is the part most commonly used in herbal remedies.

2. LOCATION: While native to parts of Asia, Astragalus has been cultivated in many other countries, including the United States, where conditions for growing are similar to its native habitat.

3. GROWING CONDITIONS: Astragalus thrives in sandy, well-drained soil under full sun. It prefers slightly alkaline soil and is quite drought-resistant once established. It typically requires at least five years of growth before the roots are harvested for medicinal use.

4. TRADITIONAL USES: Traditionally, Astragalus has been used in Chinese medicine to boost the immune system, prevent colds and upper respiratory infections, and to increase overall vitality. It's also used to support heart health and to manage blood sugar levels.

5. SCIENTIFIC BENEFITS: The roots of Astragalus are rich in saponins, flavonoids, and polysaccharides. These compounds are believed to have immunostimulant, hepatoprotective, and antiviral properties. Research suggests that Astragalus can help enhance the body's resistance to infections, support cardiac function, and act as an antioxidant, protecting cells against damage.

6. METAPHYSICAL USES: In metaphysical practices, Astragalus is often used for protection and energy enhancement. It is believed to increase one's life force or Qi, which can strengthen the body's natural defenses and help clear energy blockages. It's commonly used in practices to enhance stamina and resilience.

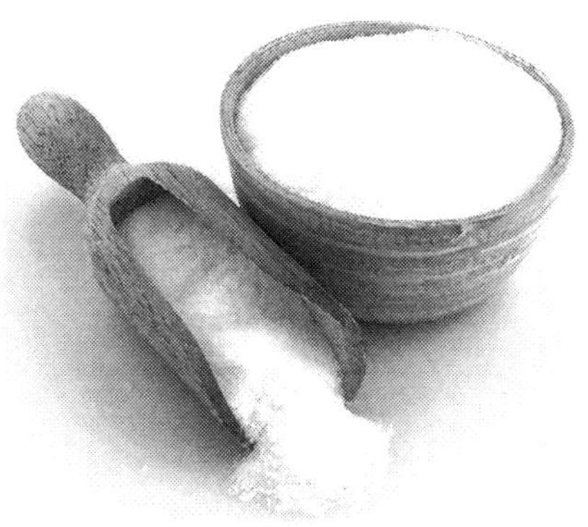

BAKING SODA

(SODIUM BICARBONATE)

is a widely used compound in cooking and various other applications.

1. DESCRIPTION: Baking soda is a white crystalline powder that is naturally alkaline, or basic in nature. It's known for its versatile properties which include leavening in baking, odor neutralization, and mild abrasive qualities.

2. LOCATION: Sodium bicarbonate occurs naturally in mineral springs but most commercially available baking soda is manufactured through chemical processes.

3. GROWING CONDITIONS: As it is a chemical compound, sodium bicarbonate does not have growing conditions per se, but it is produced through a synthetic process typically involving sodium carbonate or soda ash.

4. TRADITIONAL USES: Traditionally, baking soda has been used primarily in baking as a leavening agent where it reacts with acidic components to produce carbon dioxide gas, which causes dough to rise. It's also used in traditional household cleaning practices for scrubbing and as a deodorizing agent.

5. SCIENTIFIC BENEFITS: Baking soda is noted for its ability to neutralize acids, making it effective in relieving heartburn, indigestion, and upset stomach. It's also used in oral care as a toothpaste for its mild abrasive properties which help in removing plaque from teeth. Additionally, baking soda is used in certain dermatological applications to soothe itchy skin and relieve minor skin irritations.

6. METAPHYSICAL USES: In metaphysical practices, baking soda is often used for purification and cleansing rituals. It is believed to cleanse both physical spaces and spiritual energies, acting as a grounding agent that absorbs negative energies and promotes a clear, positive environment.

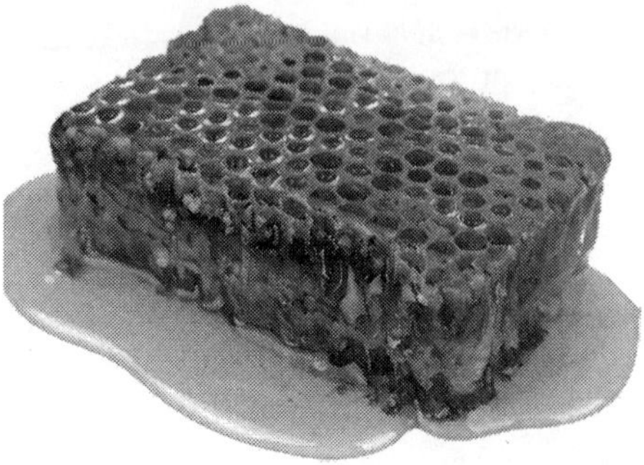

BEE PROPOLIS

also known as bee glue, is a resinous mixture that honey bees produce by mixing their saliva and beeswax with exudate gathered from tree buds, sap flows, or other botanical sources.

1. DESCRIPTION: Propolis is a sticky, greenish-brown product used by bees to coat and seal their hives, protecting it against external contaminants. It has a distinctive aromatic smell and varies in color, usually depending on its botanical source.

2. LOCATION: Bee propolis is found in bee hives around the world. The exact composition of propolis can vary significantly depending on the location of the hive and the specific trees and flowers to which the bees have access.

3. GROWING CONDITIONS: As a natural bee product, propolis is not grown but rather collected. The environmental conditions affecting its composition include the type of vegetation available to bees in the area, climate, and the health of the bee colony.

4. TRADITIONAL USES: Traditionally, propolis has been used in folk medicine since ancient times. It has been applied as an antimicrobial, antifungal, and anti-inflammatory agent. Propolis tinctures and extracts are used in various cultures to heal wounds, soothe sore throats, and improve skin conditions.

5. SCIENTIFIC BENEFITS: Propolis is rich in flavonoids and phenolic compounds, which contribute to its potent antioxidant properties. It has been studied for its antimicrobial properties which make it beneficial in fighting infections and boosting the immune system. It's also used in oral health products to prevent dental cavities and as an anti-inflammatory agent to treat diseases such as arthritis.

6. METAPHYSICAL USES: In metaphysical practices, propolis is used for spiritual protection and healing. It is believed to provide a barrier against negative energies and is used in spells and rituals to seal intentions and safeguard an individual's aura.

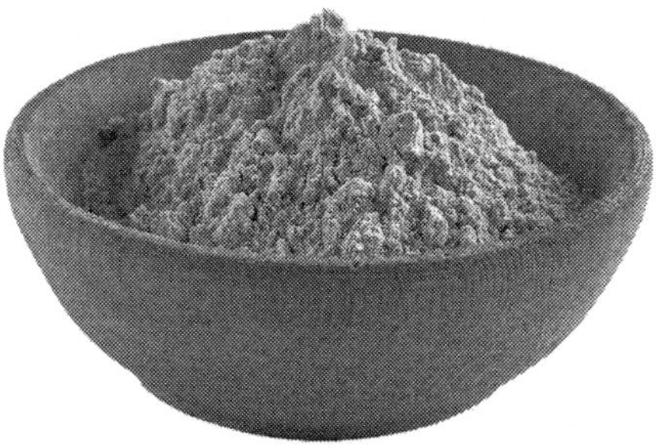

BENTONITE CLAY

also known as Montmorillonite clay, is a type of absorbent clay that typically forms from weathering of volcanic ash, most often in the presence of water.

1. DESCRIPTION: Bentonite clay is composed mainly of montmorillonite, a group of minerals, and is known for its ability to swell and absorb large quantities of water. Its color can range from light gray to cream, depending on its composition and impurities.

2. LOCATION: Major deposits of bentonite clay are found in Fort Benton, Wyoming, which is its namesake. Additionally, significant quantities are found in the Montmorillon region of France, Italy, and parts of Greece, as well as in the United States in places like Arizona and Texas.

3. GROWING CONDITIONS: Bentonite clay is mined from the earth where it forms naturally from the chemical weathering of volcanic ash.

4. TRADITIONAL USES: Traditionally, bentonite clay has been used for health and purification purposes. It has been consumed orally to detoxify the body, applied externally as a mud pack or in baths, and used in the skin care industry to make clay masks, which help to remove toxins and impurities from the skin.

5. SCIENTIFIC BENEFITS: Bentonite clay has a high concentration of minerals including silica, calcium, magnesium, sodium, iron, and potassium. It is known for its ability to absorb and remove toxins, heavy metals, impurities, and chemicals from the body, making it a popular ingredient in detox regimens. Its adsorptive properties are also beneficial for skin health, helping to clear up acne and provide a deep cleanse for pores.

6. METAPHYSICAL USES: In metaphysical practices, bentonite clay is used for purification, grounding, and protection. It is thought to help in removing negative energies from the physical and etheric bodies, and it's often used in rituals to promote emotional healing and balance.

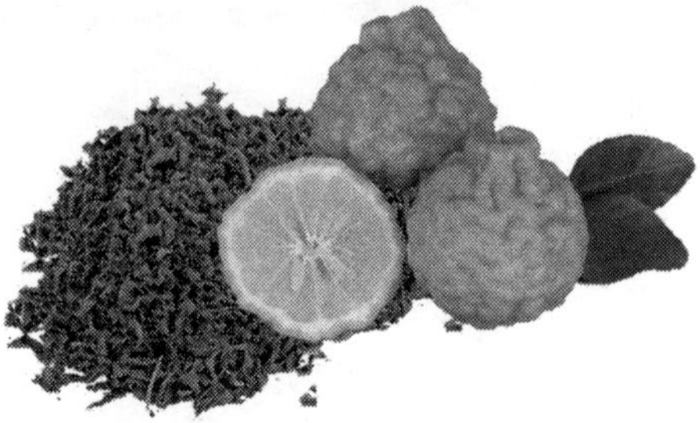

BLACK TEA WITH BERGAMOT

often recognized as Earl Grey tea, is a blend of black tea leaves flavored with oil extracted from the rind of the bergamot orange, a fragrant citrus fruit.

1. DESCRIPTION: This tea is characterized by its distinct flavor profile-black tea provides a robust, deep base, while bergamot offers a bright, citrusy, and somewhat floral aroma. The combination results in a uniquely fragrant and refreshing cup of tea.
2. LOCATION: Black tea is primarily grown in countries like India, Sri Lanka, and China, while bergamot oranges are mainly cultivated in Italy, particularly in the Calabria region, which is known for producing nearly 80% of the world's supply.
3. GROWING CONDITIONS:
   - o Black Tea: Thrives in tropical and subtropical climates with high humidity, rich soil, and at elevations ranging from sea level to 2,000 meters. It requires ample rainfall and prefers acidic soils.
   - o Bergamot: Grows in a Mediterranean climate, needing full sun and well-drained soil. It is less tolerant of extreme cold or frost than other citrus fruits.
4. TRADITIONAL USES: Earl Grey tea has been a popular choice in British tea culture since the early 19th century. It's commonly enjoyed in the afternoon with a slice of cake or biscuits. The tea is also used as a refreshing drink, either hot or iced, and is sometimes incorporated into culinary recipes like cakes, sauces, and cocktails for its distinctive flavor.
5. SCIENTIFIC BENEFITS: Black tea is rich in antioxidants known as polyphenols, which can help reduce inflammation and the risk of chronic diseases. Bergamot contains compounds like flavonoids that may help manage cholesterol levels and support overall cardiovascular health. The aroma of bergamot has been noted for its calming effect, potentially aiding in stress relief and mood improvement.
6. METAPHYSICAL USES: In metaphysical practices, Earl Grey tea is often used for clarity, spiritual awakening, and mood enhancement. Bergamot's citrus scent is believed to uplift the spirit, clear the mind, and release negative energy. It's frequently used in rituals that focus on balance, harmony, and the enhancement of one's emotional well-being.

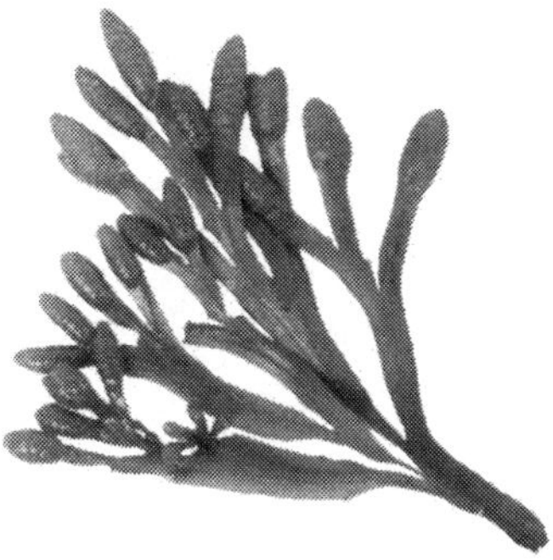

BLADDERWRACK

(FUCUS VESICULOSUS)

is a type of brown seaweed commonly found along the coasts of the North Sea, the western Baltic Sea, and the Atlantic and Pacific Oceans. It's one of the most abundant forms of kelp.

1. DESCRIPTION: Bladderwrack is easily identifiable by its olive-brown or green color, with a thallus (the body of seaweed) divided into branching strips with rounded air-filled bladders that help it float near the ocean's surface. These bladders are typically paired on either side of a central midrib.

2. LOCATION: This seaweed is prevalent in cooler waters along the coasts of many countries, including the United States, Canada, and the United Kingdom. It grows attached to rocky substrates in tidal zones where water depths allow sufficient light for photosynthesis.

3. GROWING CONDITIONS: Bladderwrack thrives in nutrient-rich, cold marine environments. It attaches itself to rocks and other hard substrates in intertidal zones up to shallow subtidal areas, tolerating a range of wave exposures and salinities.

4. TRADITIONAL USES: Historically, bladderwrack has been used as a source of iodine, an essential nutrient for thyroid function. It has also been used in traditional medicine for weight loss, arthritis, joint pain, and digestion due to its high content of fiber and essential minerals.

5. SCIENTIFIC BENEFITS: Bladderwrack is rich in iodine, which is vital for thyroid health, helping to regulate hormones responsible for controlling metabolism, energy, and growth. It also contains fucoidan, a type of complex carbohydrate that is anti-inflammatory, anti-tumor, and antioxidant. Bladderwrack has been studied for its potential in treating obesity, arthritis, and other inflammatory conditions due to its high mineral content and bioactive compounds.

6. METAPHYSICAL USES: In metaphysical practices, bladderwrack is used for money, protection, and sea spells. It is believed to bring abundance, prosperity, and good luck. Additionally, it is used in rituals to invoke the protective and nurturing qualities of the sea, often utilized in amulets or as part of ritual baths.

BLUE LOTUS

(NYMPHAEA CAERULEA)

also known as the Egyptian lotus or sacred blue lily, is a water lily native to Egypt and certain parts of Asia. It holds significant cultural and spiritual importance in various ancient civilizations, particularly in ancient Egypt.

BLUE LOTUS INFUSED MCT OIL

LAVENDER DREAMS OF A BLUE LOTUS

1. DESCRIPTION: The Blue Lotus features star-shaped flowers with vibrant blue petals and a yellow center. The flowers sit atop the water surface, supported by long stems that connect to their roots in the mud of pond or river bottoms. The leaves are broad and round, floating on the water's surface.

2. LOCATION: Originally found along the Nile and other parts of East Africa, it has spread to other warm regions including parts of Southeast Asia and the Indian subcontinent.

3. GROWING CONDITIONS: This aquatic plant thrives in muddy, shallow waters with full sunlight. It requires warm temperatures to flourish and is often found in ponds, river edges, and other calm freshwater environments.

4. TRADITIONAL USES: Historically, the Blue Lotus was used in ancient Egyptian ceremonies for its psychoactive and aphrodisiac properties, believed to induce an altered state of consciousness. It was commonly used in religious rituals to promote divine connection, and it was also celebrated as a symbol of the universe, rebirth, and beauty.

5. SCIENTIFIC BENEFITS: The Blue Lotus contains compounds like nuciferine and aporphine, which are known for their psychoactive properties. These compounds can act as natural sedatives, helping to relieve stress and anxiety, promote relaxation, and enhance sleep quality. There are also claims of its antioxidant properties, though these are less documented.

6. METAPHYSICAL USES: In metaphysical practices, the Blue Lotus is often used to enhance meditation, spiritual awareness, and psychic abilities. It is believed to be a spiritual enhancer, aiding in the opening of the third eye, promoting lucid dreaming, and encouraging spiritual growth.

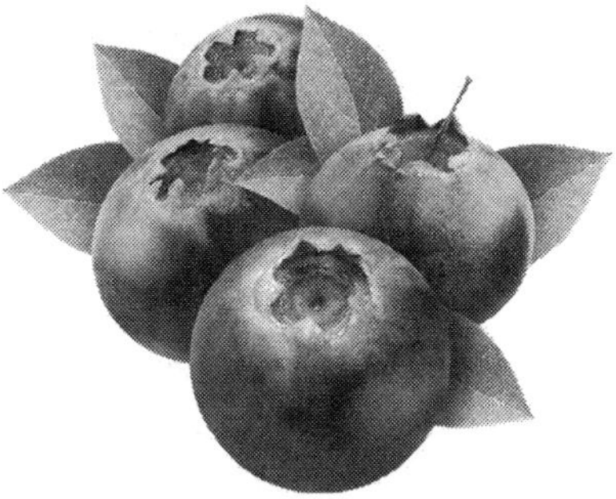

BLUEBERRY

(GENUS VACCINIUM)

is a fruit-bearing shrub that is known for its delicious and nutritious berries. It's native to North America but is now grown globally.

1. DESCRIPTION: Blueberries are small, round fruits that typically have a deep blue to purple-black color with a silvery bloom. The bushes are perennial flowering plants that can range in size from 10 centimeters to 4 meters in height, depending on the variety. They have bell-shaped flowers, which mature into the juicy berries we eat.
2. LOCATION: Originally from North America, blueberries are now cultivated in regions with similar climates around the world, including Europe, Australia, and South America. They thrive in areas with cool winters and moderate summers.
3. GROWING CONDITIONS: Blueberries prefer acidic soils with a pH between 4 and 5.5. They require well-drained, moist soil rich in organic matter. Full sunlight is ideal, although they can tolerate partial shade. They are sensitive to waterlogged roots and require consistent irrigation during the growing season.
4. TRADITIONAL USES: Traditionally, blueberries have been eaten fresh or used in a variety of dishes such as pies, muffins, and jams. Native American tribes used blueberries in medicinal practices, and the fruit was dried and added to soups and stews or ground into a powder.
5. SCIENTIFIC BENEFITS: Blueberries are highly regarded for their antioxidant properties, primarily due to their high levels of anthocyanins, which can help combat oxidative stress and inflammation. Studies suggest that regular consumption of blueberries may improve heart health, aid in maintaining brain function, and reduce the risk of type 2 diabetes. They are also rich in dietary fiber, vitamins C and K, and manganese.
6. METAPHYSICAL USES: In metaphysical practices, blueberries are associated with protection and peace. They are used in rituals to bring calm and tranquility to the home and to safeguard against negative energies. Eating blueberries is believed to enhance clarity of thought and purity of spirit.

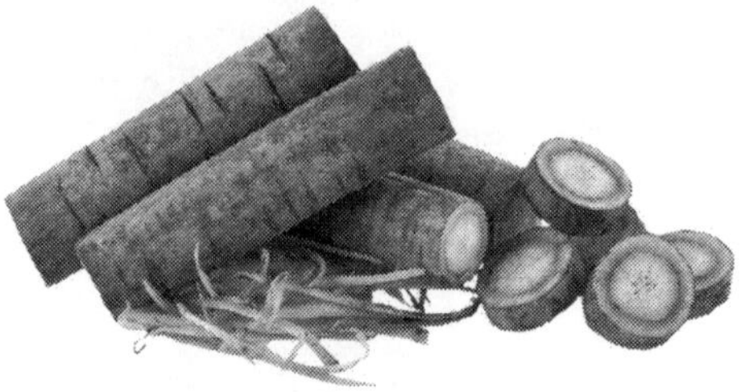

BURDOCK ROOT

(ARCTIUM LAPPA)

is a versatile plant known for its large, woolly leaves and distinctive burrs, which attach to animals and clothing for seed dispersal. The root is edible and highly valued both in culinary and herbal medicine contexts.

1. DESCRIPTION: The root is thick, fibrous, and typically brownish on the outside with a white flesh inside. It can grow up to several feet in length and has a sweet, earthy flavor when cooked.

2. LOCATION: Originally native to Europe and Asia, burdock is now widespread across the United States and many other countries, thriving in temperate regions.

3. GROWING CONDITIONS: It prefers rich, well-drained soil, although it can grow in a variety of soil types. Burdock is not particularly fussy about sunlight and can grow in both full sun and partial shade.

4. TRADITIONAL USES: In traditional medicine, particularly in Asia, burdock root is used to purify blood, enhance liver function, and as a natural diuretic. In Japan, it is commonly eaten as a vegetable, known as gobo, and is featured in dishes like kinpira gobo (sautéed burdock with carrots).

5. SCIENTIFIC BENEFITS: Rich in important antioxidants, burdock root is believed to help remove toxins from the bloodstream. It also contains inulin, a prebiotic that may improve gut health. Its anti-inflammatory properties are useful for skin health, helping to treat conditions like acne and eczema.

6. METAPHYSICAL USES: Burdock root is used in various spiritual practices for protection and cleansing. It is thought to be particularly powerful for warding off negative energies and is used in protective spells and incantations.

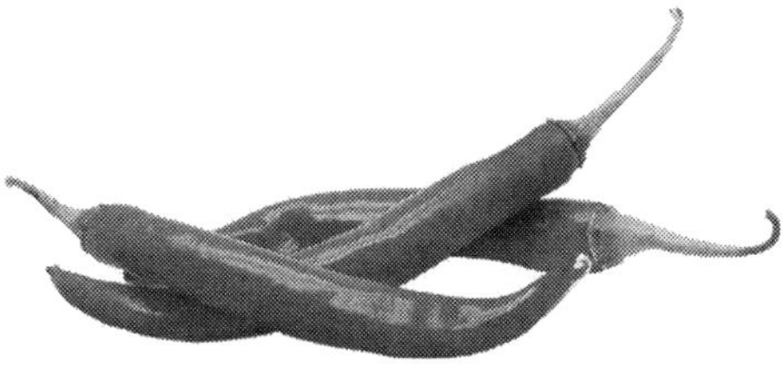

CAYENNE PEPPER

(CAPSICUM ANNUUM)

is a hot chili pepper used to flavor dishes and for various health benefits. It is recognized by its long, thin, and bright red appearance.

1. DESCRIPTION: The peppers are typically dried and ground to produce a fine red powder, but they are also used fresh in cooking. The spice derived from these peppers is known for its pungent taste and vibrant red color.

2. LOCATION: Native to the tropical regions of the Americas, cayenne peppers are now grown globally in various warm climates that can support their growth.

3. GROWING CONDITIONS: These peppers prefer a warm, moist environment and full sunlight. They grow best in temperatures between 70°F and 85°F and require well-drained, nutrient-rich soil.

4. TRADITIONAL USES: In addition to culinary uses, cayenne is traditionally used in herbal medicine to help with digestion, improve circulation, and relieve muscle and joint pain due to its anti-inflammatory properties.

5. SCIENTIFIC BENEFITS: The key component of cayenne pepper, capsaicin, has been studied for its effects on reducing pain and inflammation, boosting metabolism, and even as a potential anticancer agent. It also helps to clear congestion by thinning mucus.

6. METAPHYSICAL USES: In metaphysical practices, cayenne is often used to add power to protective charms, to cleanse negativity from a space, and to drive away unwanted influences. It is also used to enhance the effectiveness of spells by adding an element of "heat" or urgency.

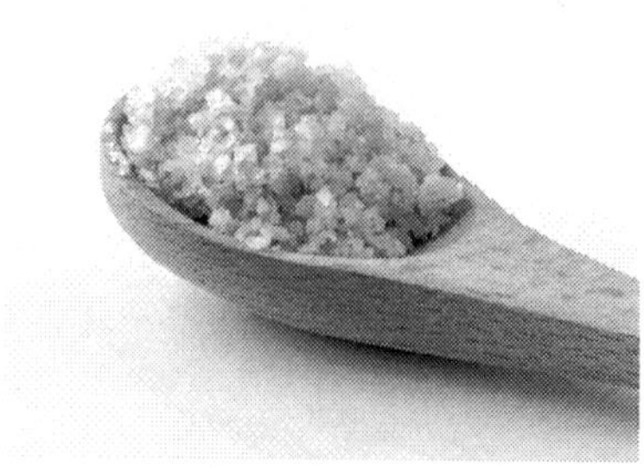

CELTIC SEA SALT

is a type of sea salt that is harvested using traditional Celtic methods, primarily from the coastal areas of France. The salt is known for its moist, grey appearance, which it retains from the clay found in salt flats.

1. DESCRIPTION: This salt is unrefined and contains a bit of residual moisture, which helps preserve its rich mineral content. Its color can range from light grey to almost black, depending on the harvesting area and methods.

2. LOCATION: Celtic Sea Salt is primarily harvested in the Brittany region of France, where the natural clay and sand create a unique filtration system as the sea water evaporates.

3. GROWING CONDITIONS: As a naturally occurring mineral, Celtic Sea Salt is collected from tidal pools that are allowed to evaporate under the sun. The salt is then hand-raked in a traditional method that preserves its natural state and mineral content.

4. TRADITIONAL USES: Traditionally, Celtic Sea Salt has been used for its flavor in cooking and preserving food. It is also valued in traditional health practices for its trace minerals, which are believed to aid hydration and balance electrolytes.

5. SCIENTIFIC BENEFITS: Celtic Sea Salt is touted for its lower sodium and higher mineral content compared to regular table salt. It contains numerous trace minerals, including magnesium, calcium, and potassium, which are essential for maintaining proper health. These minerals can help in fluid balance, promoting heart health, and preventing muscle cramps.

6. METAPHYSICAL USES: In metaphysical practices, Celtic Sea Salt is often used for purification and protection rituals. It is believed to cleanse spaces of negative energies and to create barriers against external influences. It's also used in bath rituals for detoxification and grounding.

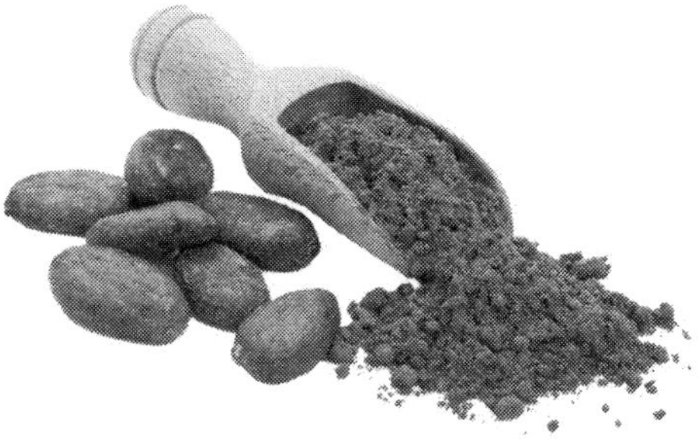

CEREMONIAL GRADE CACAO

is a high-quality cacao used primarily for spiritual and ceremonial purposes. It is less processed than commercial cacao or cocoa products, retaining more of its natural nutrients.

1. DESCRIPTION: This form of cacao is typically made from whole cacao beans that are minimally processed to preserve their natural properties. It often comes in blocks or paste and has a rich, deep chocolate flavor and aroma.

2. LOCATION: Ceremonial grade cacao is primarily sourced from cacao beans grown in Central and South America, particularly in countries like Peru, Ecuador, and Guatemala, where cacao cultivation has deep cultural and historical significance.

3. GROWING CONDITIONS: Cacao trees thrive in the humid tropical climates of the rainforest. They require a mixture of shade and humidity, typically growing under the canopy of taller trees. The soil must be rich in organic materials and well-drained.

4. TRADITIONAL USES: Traditionally, cacao has been used in various indigenous ceremonies, often as a sacred beverage that promotes connection, community, and spiritual well-being. It was considered a gift from the gods in many Mesoamerican cultures.

5. SCIENTIFIC BENEFITS: Ceremonial grade cacao is rich in antioxidants, particularly flavonoids, which are known to help reduce inflammation and improve heart health. It also contains a significant amount of magnesium, which can support muscle and nerve function, and theobromine, a natural stimulant that can enhance alertness and mood.

6. METAPHYSICAL USES: In metaphysical practices, cacao is used to open the heart chakra and enhance meditation. It is considered a powerful tool for reaching deeper emotional and spiritual levels, facilitating inner healing, creativity, and a deeper connection with oneself and others.

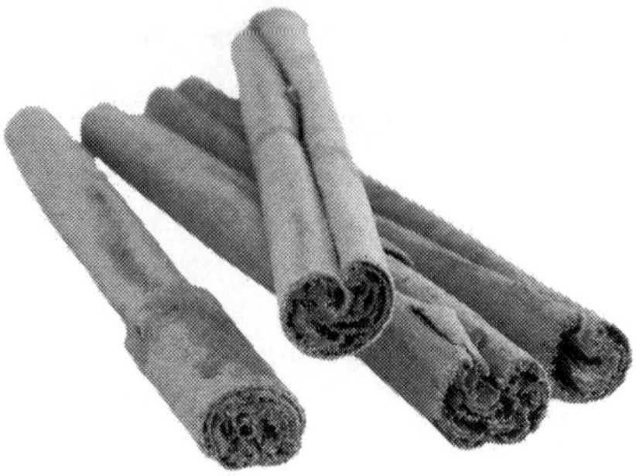

CEYLON CINNAMON

also known as "true cinnamon," is a highly prized variety of cinnamon that originates from the Cinnamomum verum tree.

1. DESCRIPTION: Ceylon cinnamon is lighter in color and has a finer, less dense, and more crumbly texture compared to the more common Cassia cinnamon. Its flavor is also considered to be more delicate and slightly sweeter.

2. LOCATION: Native to Sri Lanka (formerly known as Ceylon), it is also cultivated in parts of India, Madagascar, Brazil, and the Caribbean.

3. GROWING CONDITIONS: Ceylon cinnamon trees thrive in warm, humid climates with well-drained, sandy soils. They are typically grown in partial to full shade and require consistent moisture for optimal growth.

4. TRADITIONAL USES: Traditionally, Ceylon cinnamon has been used both as a spice in cooking and baking and in traditional medicine for its health benefits. It has been used to treat colds, flu, and digestive issues and as a natural preservative due to its antibacterial properties.

5. SCIENTIFIC BENEFITS: Ceylon cinnamon is rich in antioxidants, which help protect the body from oxidative stress and may reduce the risk of disease. It is also noted for its anti-inflammatory properties and its potential to help regulate blood sugar levels, making it beneficial for people with type 2 diabetes. Unlike Cassia cinnamon, Ceylon cinnamon contains much lower amounts of coumarin, which is safer for regular consumption.

6. METAPHYSICAL USES: In metaphysical practices, Ceylon cinnamon is used for its spiritual and protective properties. It is believed to enhance healing, promote prosperity and success, and purify spaces. It is also used in love spells and for raising spiritual vibrations during rituals.

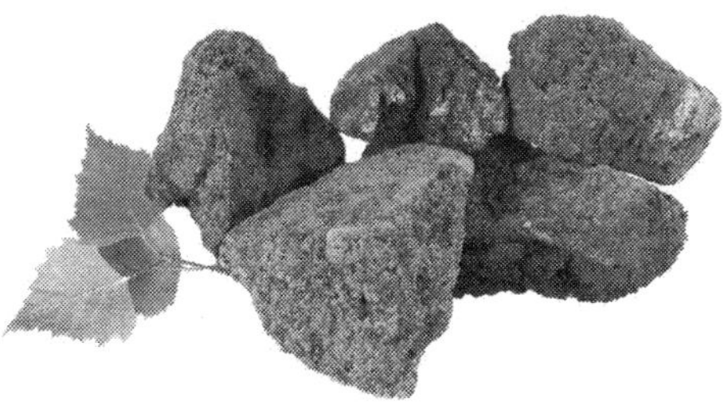

CHAGA MUSHROOM

(INONOTUS OBLIQUUS)

is a type of fungus that grows primarily on the bark of birch trees in cold climates. It is not a typical mushroom in appearance; instead, it looks more like a clump of burnt charcoal due to its black, crusty exterior. The interior is a rich brown with a somewhat woody texture.

1. DESCRIPTION: Chaga is distinguished by its irregular, lumpy form and burnt cork-like texture, which masks a rich, rusty brown interior. It is often ground into a fine powder for medicinal use.

2. LOCATION: Chaga is most commonly found in the birch forests of Russia, Korea, Eastern and Northern Europe, Northern areas of the United States, and Canada.

3. GROWING CONDITIONS: Chaga mushrooms grow best in cold climates and are predominantly found on the trunks of mature birch trees. It feeds off the lignin in birch trees and often takes years to accumulate substantial size.

4. TRADITIONAL USES: Traditionally, Chaga has been used in folk medicine, particularly in Northern Europe and Russia, for boosting immunity and overall health. It has been used to make a medicinal tea that helps with various ailments, from stomach diseases to heart ailments and diabetes.

5. SCIENTIFIC BENEFITS: Chaga is rich in antioxidants and compounds that can help reduce inflammation and support the immune system. It contains betulinic acid, which is derived from the birch trees it grows on and has been studied for its potential to inhibit cancer cell growth. Chaga is also known for its potential to lower blood sugar and cholesterol levels.

6. METAPHYSICAL USES: In metaphysical practices, Chaga is used for grounding and protection. It is believed to absorb negativity and to protect against the draining of energy. It's also used in rituals aimed at enhancing longevity and improving overall vitality.

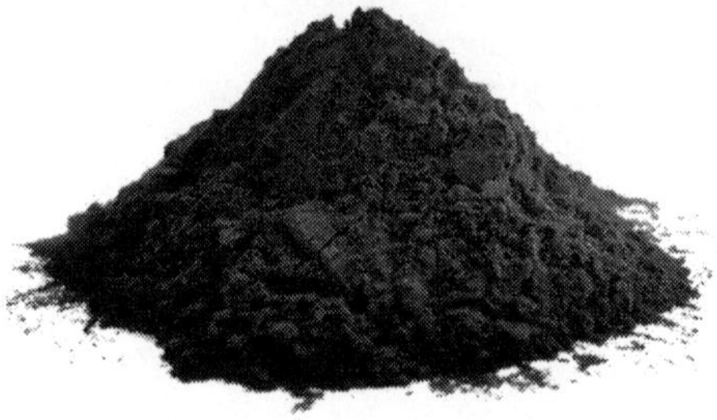

CHARCOAL

(ACTIVATED)

is a form of carbon processed to have small, low-volume pores that increase the surface area available for adsorption or chemical reactions. It's typically made from carbon-rich materials such as wood, coconut shells, or peat.

1. DESCRIPTION: Activated charcoal is a fine, odorless, black powder often used in emergency rooms to treat overdoses or poisonings, thanks to its toxin-absorbing properties. Its high degree of microporosity makes just a single gram of activated charcoal have a surface area in excess of 3,000 square meters.

2. LOCATION: As a manufactured product, activated charcoal can be produced anywhere there is an availability of carbon-rich materials, though it is commonly produced in high volumes in industrialized countries.

3. GROWING CONDITIONS: Not applicable, as activated charcoal is an engineered product derived from natural materials that are processed at high temperatures to activate the carbon.

4. TRADITIONAL USES: Traditionally, activated charcoal has been used to purify water and in medical practices to absorb toxins and drugs from the gastrointestinal tract. It is also used in air purification systems to remove odors and toxins from the air.

5. SCIENTIFIC BENEFITS: Activated charcoal is most renowned for its use in toxin absorption in cases of poisoning or drug overdoses. It helps prevent the gastrointestinal absorption of a wide variety of drugs and toxins, effectively reducing their systemic effects. It is also used in kidney health for patients suffering from chronic kidney disease, as it helps absorb waste products to reduce the burden on the kidneys.

6. METAPHYSICAL USES: In metaphysical practices, activated charcoal is used for purification and cleansing. It is believed to absorb negative energies and cleanse both physical and etheric bodies. It's often used in rituals and as a component in spells that focus on detoxifying one's life or environment.

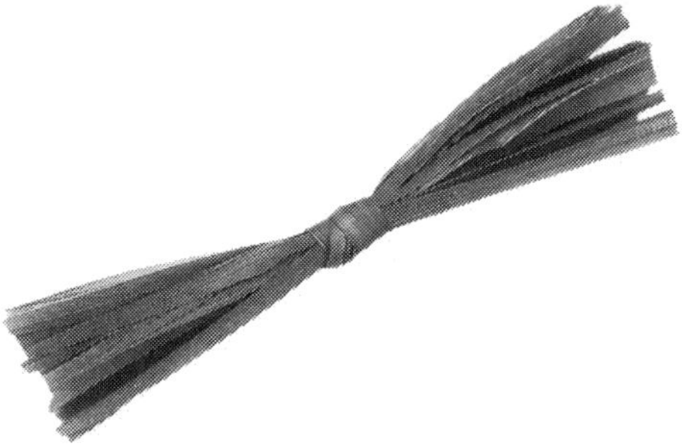

CHLORELLA

(INONOTUS OBLIQUUS)

is a single-celled green algae that is incredibly nutrient-dense and grows in freshwater bodies. It is highly regarded for its nutritional and medicinal benefits.

1. DESCRIPTION: Chlorella is a microscopic, spherical algae that is green due to its high concentration of chlorophyll. It multiplies rapidly under the right conditions and is harvested to be processed into supplements and powders.

2. LOCATION: While chlorella is native to Taiwan and Japan, it is cultivated worldwide in controlled aquatic farms to ensure purity and optimal nutrient content.

3. GROWING CONDITIONS: Chlorella requires water, light, carbon dioxide, and small amounts of minerals to grow. It thrives best in warm, sunlit, and pH-controlled water environments. Its rapid growth rate makes it a sustainable source of nutrients.

4. TRADITIONAL USES: Traditionally, chlorella has been used in health supplements for its purported detoxifying properties. It has been used to boost energy, support fat loss, and as a source of complete protein and other vitamins.

5. SCIENTIFIC BENEFITS: Chlorella is packed with nutrients, including protein, omega-3 fatty acids, vitamins B12, C, and E, and minerals such as iron and magnesium. It's particularly noted for its ability to bind with heavy metals and other toxins to facilitate their removal from the body. Additionally, it supports immune function, reduces cholesterol, and acts as an antioxidant.

6. METAPHYSICAL USES: In metaphysical practices, chlorella is used for cleansing and protection. It is believed to promote clarity of mind and physical vitality, making it a popular choice for rituals that focus on healing and energy renewal.

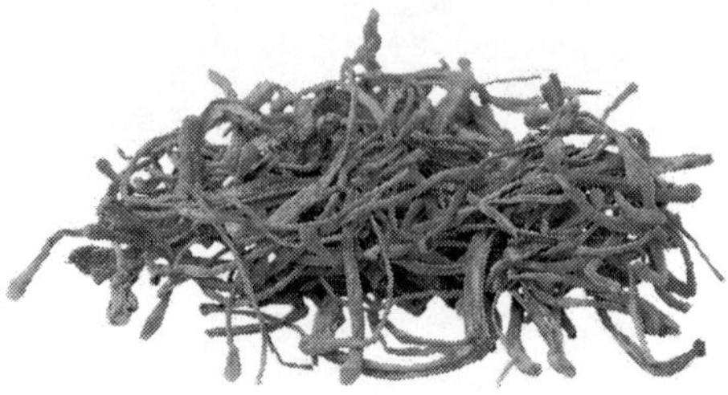

CORDYCEPS MUSHROOM

(OPHIOCORDYCEPS SINENSIS)

is a type of parasitic fungus that grows on the larvae of insects. When these fungi attack their host, they replace its tissue and sprout long, slender stems that grow outside the host's body.

1. DESCRIPTION: The mushroom consists of a long, slender fruiting body, which is usually orange or brown. It is distinct for growing out of the head of the insect host, which it has consumed from the inside out.

2. LOCATION: Cordyceps is primarily found in the high mountain regions of China, particularly in the Himalayas, but also grows in the high altitude regions of Tibet, Nepal, and Bhutan.

3. GROWING CONDITIONS: Cordyceps thrives in high altitude, cold, grassy, alpine environments where specific species of insects inhabit. The fungus starts as a spore that infects the insect host, eventually growing into a mushroom that emerges from the host's body.

4. TRADITIONAL USES: Traditionally, Cordyceps has been used in Chinese medicine for centuries for its vitality-enhancing and anti-aging properties. It is often prescribed to improve energy, appetite, stamina, libido, endurance, and sleeping patterns.

5. SCIENTIFIC BENEFITS: Cordyceps is known for its potential to increase ATP production in the body, which is the primary energy carrier in the cells. This can enhance physical performance and help fight fatigue. It also has anti-inflammatory properties, may help manage blood sugar levels, and supports heart health. Some studies indicate it might boost the immune system and have anti-aging effects.

6. METAPHYSICAL USES: In metaphysical practices, Cordyceps is often used for increasing life force and vitality. It is believed to enhance one's spiritual energy and physical stamina, making it popular in practices aimed at rejuvenation and extending one's life energy.

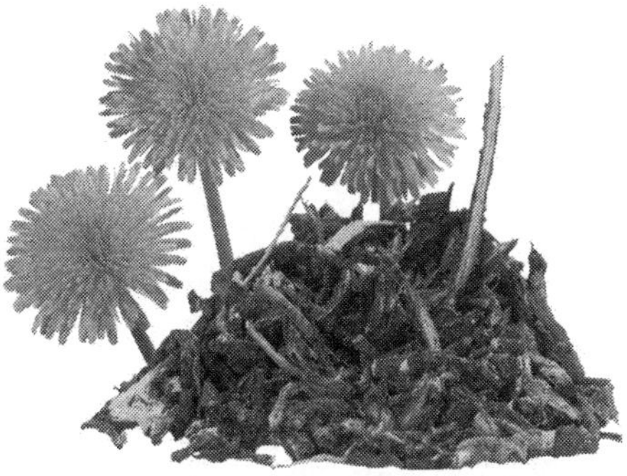

DANDELION ROOTS

come from the common dandelion plant (Taraxacum officinale), a flowering herbaceous perennial known for its bright yellow flowers and fluffy seed heads.

1. DESCRIPTION: Dandelion roots are long, dark brown on the outside and white on the inside. They are robust and deeply anchored into the soil. The roots are known for their ability to break up compacted soil and draw nutrients up from deep within the earth.

2. LOCATION: Dandelions are native to Europe and Asia but have become widespread across all temperate regions worldwide, including North America.

3. GROWING CONDITIONS: Dandelions are extremely adaptable and can grow in a wide range of conditions, but they prefer sunny locations with fertile, well-drained soil. They are resilient and can grow in poor soil as well, making them common in urban and disturbed environments.

4. TRADITIONAL USES: Traditionally, dandelion roots have been used for their medicinal properties, particularly for liver detoxification, as a diuretic, and to aid digestion. The roots are often dried, roasted, and ground into a coffee substitute or brewed into a tea.

5. SCIENTIFIC BENEFITS: Dandelion roots are rich in inulin, a type of soluble fiber that supports healthy bacteria in the gastrointestinal tract. They contain potent antioxidants that may reduce inflammation and increase antioxidant activity. Research suggests they can help regulate blood sugar and cholesterol levels, support liver health, and promote digestion.

6. METAPHYSICAL USES: In metaphysical practices, dandelion root is often used for grounding and divination. It is believed to promote psychic abilities and clarity of thought, and is used in spells and rituals for manifesting wishes and calling forth spirits.

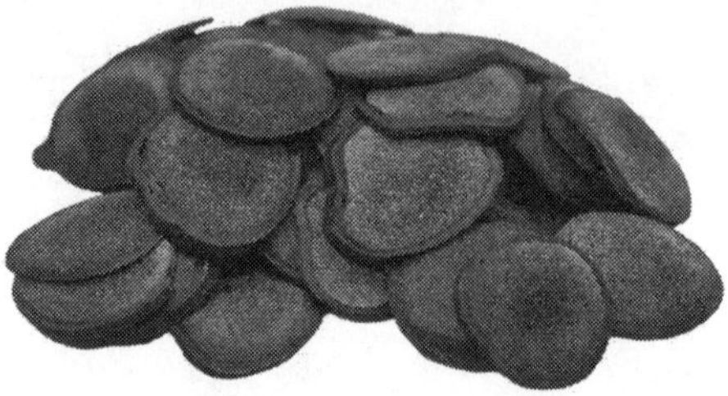

DEER ANTLER

also known as velvet antler, refers to the antlers of deer during their phase of rapid growth, which is covered in a soft, velvety skin. It is harvested primarily from male deer, without harming the animal, as the antlers regrow every year.

1. DESCRIPTION: Deer antlers are bony structures that can regenerate annually. In their growth phase, they are soft, covered in a fine velvet-like fur, and rich in blood vessels and nerves.

2. LOCATION: While deer antlers can be harvested in many countries where deer are found, major producers include New Zealand, China, Russia, and Canada.

3. GROWING CONDITIONS: Not applicable, as deer antlers are an animal product.

4. TRADITIONAL USES: Traditionally, deer antler has been used in Chinese medicine to enhance bone health, support joint mobility, and improve overall vitality and endurance. It is typically ground into a powder and consumed in capsule form or as a tea.

5. SCIENTIFIC BENEFITS: Deer antler velvet is rich in amino acids, growth hormones, and minerals. It is believed to promote strength and endurance, improve the way the immune system works, and counter the effects of stress. It is also noted for its use in accelerating recovery from injuries related to exercise.

6. METAPHYSICAL USES: In metaphysical practices, deer antler is used for its growth and regenerative properties. It is believed to symbolize regeneration and spiritual enlightenment. Practitioners may use it in rituals that focus on healing, growth, or spiritual rebirth.

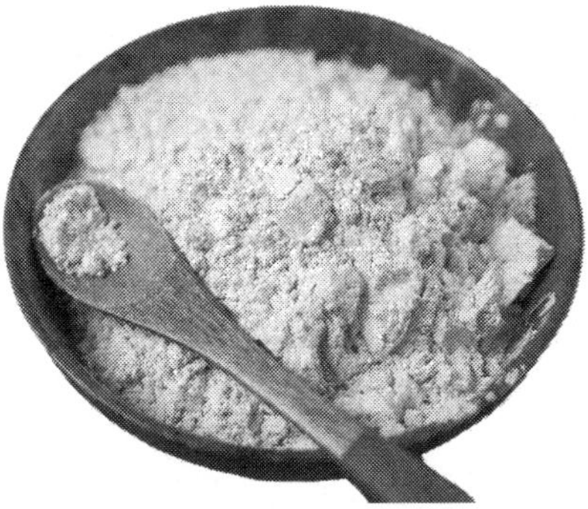

DIATOMACEOUS EARTH

(DE)

is a naturally occurring, soft, siliceous sedimentary rock that is easily crumbled into a fine white to off-white powder. It is composed of the fossilized remains of diatoms, a type of hard-shelled algae.

1. DESCRIPTION: Diatomaceous earth is a fine, abrasive powder with a mildly gritty texture. It is very light due to its high porosity and appears off-white or grey in color.

2. LOCATION: Significant deposits of diatomaceous earth can be found in the United States, especially in Nevada and parts of California, as well as in France and Russia.

3. GROWING CONDITIONS: Not applicable, as diatomaceous earth is a mineral product formed from fossilized water plants over millions of years.

4. TRADITIONAL USES: Traditionally, DE has been used as a filtering aid, for pest control, and as a mild abrasive in products like toothpaste and metal polish. It is also used in agriculture for natural insect control.

5. SCIENTIFIC BENEFITS: Diatomaceous earth is highly valued for its ability to kill insects by dehydrating them; it works mechanically rather than chemically, making it a non-toxic choice. For human consumption, food-grade DE is sometimes used as a source of silica, which is important for bone, skin, and hair health. It is also used to detoxify the body by binding with toxins and heavy metals and removing them from the system.

6. METAPHYSICAL USES: In metaphysical practices, diatomaceous earth is used for purification and protection. It is believed to absorb negative energies much like it absorbs toxins and is often used in cleansing rituals to purify physical spaces.

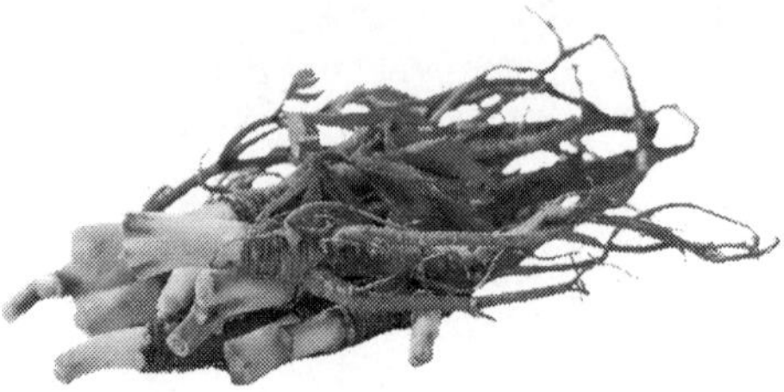

DONG QUAI

(ANGELICA SINENSIS)

also known as Chinese Angelica, is a perennial herb native to China. It is highly regarded in traditional Chinese medicine, often referred to as the "female ginseng" due to its benefits for women's health.

1. DESCRIPTION: Dong Quai has smooth purplish stems and umbrella-shaped clusters of white flowers. The medicinal part of the plant is its root, which is thick, branched, and has a sweet, pungent aroma.

2. LOCATION: While native to China, Dong Quai is also cultivated in Japan and Korea, and has been adapted to Western herbal practices.

3. GROWING CONDITIONS: Dong Quai thrives in cool and damp high-altitude regions in China. It prefers well-drained, moist, rich soil and partial shade.

4. TRADITIONAL USES: Traditionally, Dong Quai has been used to support female reproductive health, alleviate menstrual cramps, and balance hormones. It is also used to improve circulation, treat anemia, and boost energy levels.

5. SCIENTIFIC BENEFITS: Dong Quai contains compounds that may help to balance estrogen levels and support menstrual health. It is also known for its anti-inflammatory and antioxidant properties. Studies suggest that it can improve blood flow and promote heart health, although more research is needed to fully understand its effects.

6. METAPHYSICAL USES: In metaphysical practices, Dong Quai is used to harmonize and strengthen the female reproductive system. It is often utilized in rituals aimed at healing feminine energy and promoting emotional balance.

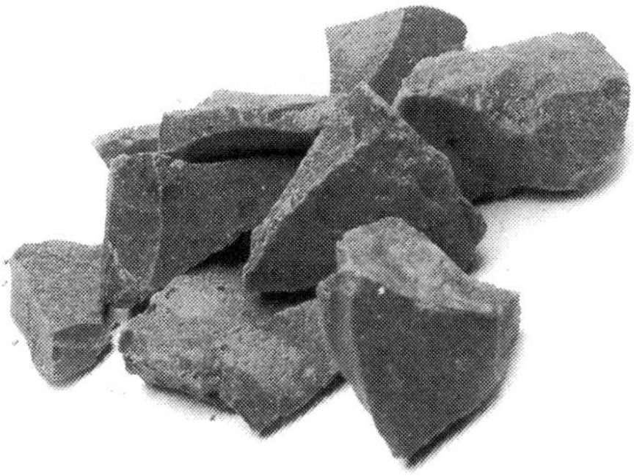

DRAGON'S BLOOD RESIN

is a natural resin obtained from various plant species, predominantly the Croton, Dracaena, Daemonorops, and Pterocarpus genera. It is named for its rich red color, which resembles the color of dragon's blood.

1. DESCRIPTION: The resin is dark red and forms hardened chunks or can be powdered. It has a distinct, slightly sweet and spicy aroma.

2. LOCATION: Dragon's blood plants are found in different regions depending on the species. Dracaena and Daemonorops species are primarily found in tropical regions of Southeast Asia, the Canary Islands, and parts of Africa. Pterocarpus species are native to South America.

3. GROWING CONDITIONS: The various plants that produce Dragon's Blood thrive in tropical climates with ample rainfall and humidity. Each species has specific environmental preferences related to its native habitat.

4. TRADITIONAL USES: Historically, Dragon's Blood resin has been used in medicine, varnishes, and incense. Medicinally, it has been applied topically to heal wounds and taken internally for digestive and respiratory issues. It is also used in traditional dyeing and painting for its vibrant color.

5. SCIENTIFIC BENEFITS: Dragon's Blood resin is rich in protective antioxidant compounds, which can help fight free radicals and repair tissue damage. It has anti-inflammatory properties and is used in various skin care products to promote healing of the skin. Research has also indicated antimicrobial properties, making it useful in preventing infections.

6. METAPHYSICAL USES: In metaphysical practices, Dragon's Blood resin is used for protection, increasing power, and purification. It is commonly used in rituals to clear negative energy, enhance personal power, and protect spaces. It is also believed to enhance love and sexual potency.

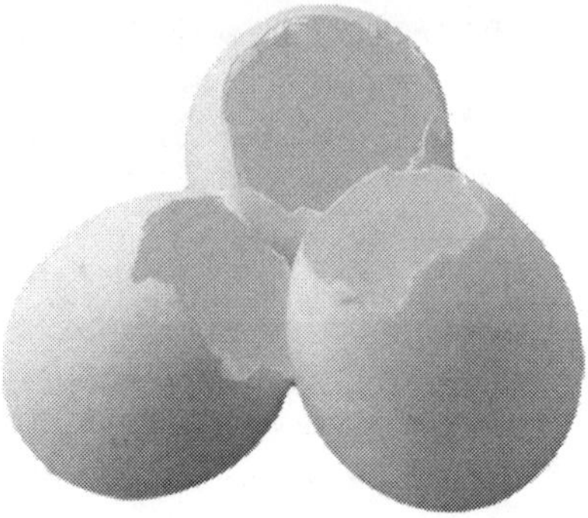

EGG SHELLS

are the outer covering of eggs, produced by birds, primarily chickens. They are composed mostly of calcium carbonate and have a semi-permeable membrane, which allows air and moisture to pass through.

1. DESCRIPTION: Egg shells are usually white or brown, depending on the breed of the chicken, and are hard and brittle. The shell's surface is covered with as many as 17,000 tiny pores.

2. LOCATION: They are a byproduct of the global poultry industry.

3. GROWING CONDITIONS: Egg shells are a by-product of egg-laying birds, primarily chickens, which are raised worldwide under various conditions.

4. TRADITIONAL USES: Traditionally, crushed egg shells have been used as a natural calcium supplement in gardening to enrich soil or mixed into animal feed. They are also used in home remedies for minor skin irritations and in arts and crafts for decoration.

5. SCIENTIFIC BENEFITS: Egg shells are primarily composed of calcium carbonate, a form of calcium that is easily absorbed by the body. They can be used as a natural calcium supplement when finely ground. Research suggests that eggshell powder can help prevent and treat osteoporosis when taken with vitamin D and magnesium.

6. METAPHYSICAL USES: In metaphysical practices, egg shells, often ground into a powder called "cascarilla," are used for protection and purification. They are commonly used in spiritual baths, to mark protective symbols, or to line the perimeter of a space to protect it from negative energy.

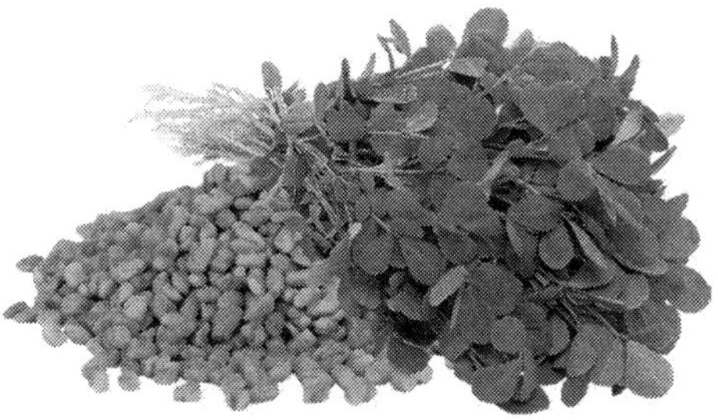

FENUGREEK SEEDS

come from the Fenugreek plant (Trigonella foenum-graecum), an herb native to the Mediterranean region, southern Europe, and western Asia.

1. DESCRIPTION: Fenugreek seeds are small, hard, and yellowish-brown. They have a strong, sweet aroma, somewhat similar to maple syrup, and a bitter taste.

2. LOCATION: While originally from the Mediterranean, fenugreek is now also cultivated in India, North Africa, and parts of the USA, particularly for its culinary and medicinal seeds.

3. GROWING CONDITIONS: Fenugreek prefers well-drained soil and a warm, sunny environment. It can thrive in a range of soil types, as long as they are not waterlogged.

4. TRADITIONAL USES: Traditionally, fenugreek seeds have been used in cooking, particularly in Indian cuisine, as a spice and flavoring agent in dishes like curries and chutneys. Medicinally, they have been used to treat digestive issues, improve cholesterol levels, and enhance lactation in nursing mothers.

5. SCIENTIFIC BENEFITS: Fenugreek seeds contain a variety of beneficial nutrients, including fiber, protein, and iron. They are known for their anti-inflammatory, antidiabetic, and anti-cholesterolemic properties. Studies suggest that fenugreek can help reduce blood sugar levels, improve glucose tolerance, and may also have a beneficial effect on triglyceride levels in the body.

6. METAPHYSICAL USES: In metaphysical practices, fenugreek seeds are used for attracting wealth, prosperity, and abundance. They are often used in money spells or carried as a charm to attract financial success.

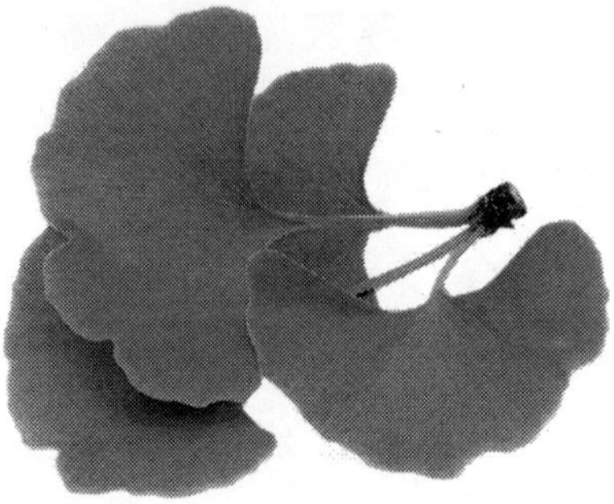

GINKGO BILOBA

also known simply as ginkgo, is one of the oldest living tree species. Its leaves are uniquely shaped and are used in various traditional remedies and modern supplements.

1. DESCRIPTION: Ginkgo leaves are fan-shaped and often split in the middle, resembling two lobes. They are bright green, turning golden yellow in the fall.

2. LOCATION: Originally native to China, ginkgo trees are now cultivated worldwide, particularly in urban areas due to their resistance to pollution and pests.

3. GROWING CONDITIONS: Ginkgo biloba thrives in well-drained soil and can tolerate a wide range of soil types and pH levels. It prefers full sun to partial shade and is notably resistant to environmental stressors.

4. TRADITIONAL USES: Traditionally, ginkgo leaves have been used to treat asthma and bronchitis and to improve cognitive function and memory. They have been used in Chinese medicine for centuries to address problems related to circulation and aging.

5. SCIENTIFIC BENEFITS: Ginkgo is best known for its potential to enhance brain health. It may improve focus, memory, and the ability to perform everyday tasks. It's thought to do this by supporting blood flow to the brain and protecting it from neuronal damage. Ginkgo also has antioxidant properties that may help fight inflammation and improve heart health and circulation.

6. METAPHYSICAL USES: In metaphysical practices, Ginkgo Biloba is used for its qualities of longevity, resilience, and strength. It is believed to aid in healing, provide mental clarity, and enhance spiritual growth and harmony. Ginkgo leaves are sometimes carried as talismans for protection or to attract healing energies.

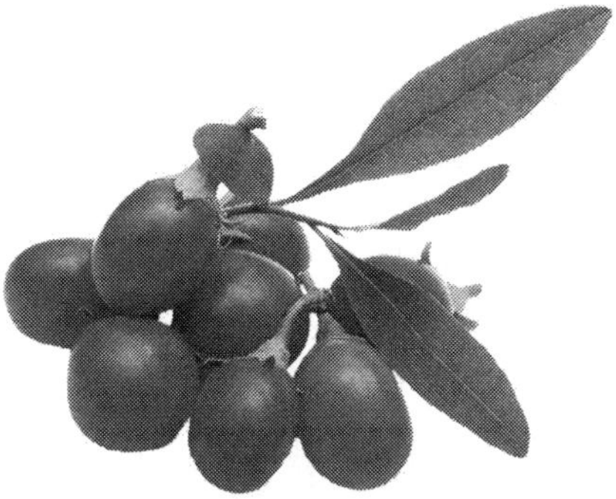

GOJI BERRIES

also known as wolfberries, are small, red fruits from the plant Lycium barbarum. They are native to Asia and are renowned for their high nutrient content and health benefits.

1. DESCRIPTION: Goji berries are bright orange-red, oblong-shaped, and typically dried for consumption. They have a slightly sweet and tart flavor and are chewy in texture when dried.

2. LOCATION: While originally from China, Mongolia, and the Tibetan Himalayas, goji berries are now cultivated in many parts of the world, including Europe and North America.

3. GROWING CONDITIONS: Goji berry plants are hardy and tolerate poor soil, drought, and harsh environments. They thrive best in alkaline soils and require full sun for optimal fruit production.

4. TRADITIONAL USES: Traditionally, goji berries have been used in Chinese medicine to enhance immune function, improve sight, protect the liver, boost sperm production, and promote longevity.

5. SCIENTIFIC BENEFITS: Goji berries are packed with antioxidants, including zeaxanthin and lycopene, which help protect the body against oxidative stress. They are also rich in vitamin C, fiber, iron, vitamin A, zinc, and antioxidants. Studies suggest that goji berries can help improve energy levels, aid in weight management, and support immune and cardiovascular health.

6. METAPHYSICAL USES: In metaphysical practices, goji berries are used to increase life force and vitality. They are believed to aid in spiritual practices by enhancing personal enlightenment and well-being. Goji berries are also used in rituals focused on health, longevity, and vision.

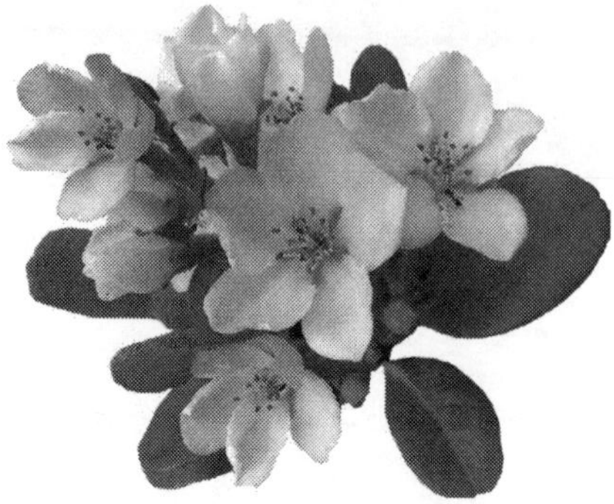

HAWTHORN

(CRATAEGUS SPECIES)

is a shrub or small tree known for its deep green leaves, white or pink flowers, and red berries. It is highly valued both for its ornamental beauty and medicinal properties.

1. DESCRIPTION: Hawthorn plants feature small, lobed leaves, clusters of fragrant white or pink flowers in the spring, followed by bright red berries in the fall. The plant can range from a dense shrub to a small tree.

2. LOCATION: Hawthorn is native to temperate regions of Europe, North America, and Asia. It is commonly found in woodland areas, along roadsides, and in hedgerows.

3. GROWING CONDITIONS: Hawthorn thrives in well-drained soil, under full sun to partial shade. It is adaptable to different soil types and environmental conditions, making it a hardy species.

4. TRADITIONAL USES: Traditionally, hawthorn has been used to treat heart-related conditions, improve circulation, and control high blood pressure and cholesterol. The leaves, flowers, and berries are all used in herbal medicine, often in the form of teas, extracts, or capsules.

5. SCIENTIFIC BENEFITS: Hawthorn is best known for its use in treating cardiovascular diseases. It is believed to improve heart function, increase blood flow, and stabilize heart rhythm. Studies suggest that hawthorn extracts may also have antioxidant properties that help dilate blood vessels, improve blood flow, and protect the vessels from damage.

6. METAPHYSICAL USES: In metaphysical practices, hawthorn is often associated with protection and cleansing. It is used in spells and rituals to purify the heart and prepare it for spiritual growth and healing. Hawthorn is also thought to enhance intuition and promote happiness.

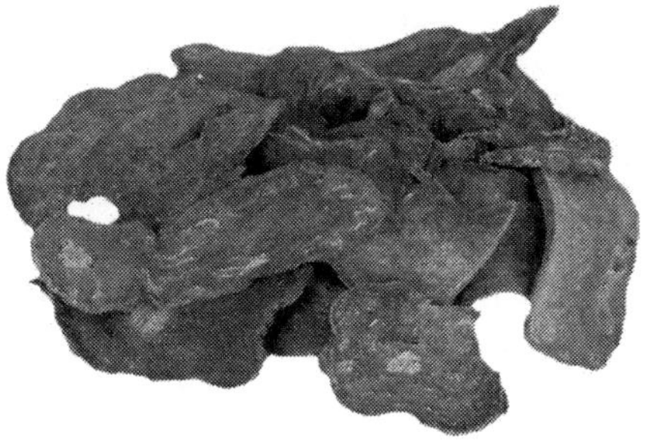

HE SHOU WU

(INONOTUS OBLIQUUS)

(also known as Fo-Ti or Polygonum multiflorum) is a revered herb in traditional Chinese medicine. It is derived from the tuberous roots of a flowering plant native to central and southern China.

1. DESCRIPTION: He Shou Wu roots are long and tuberous, often twisted together, forming a mass that is brownish on the outside and creamy white inside. The plant itself has heart-shaped leaves and either white or pink flowers.

2. LOCATION: Native to China, He Shou Wu is cultivated extensively in regions of China, Japan, and Taiwan. It thrives in their mountainous landscapes.

3. GROWING CONDITIONS: He Shou Wu prefers moist, well-drained soil in shaded or semi-shaded areas. It requires a moderate climate for optimal growth and is typically harvested after three to four years of growth for medicinal use.

4. TRADITIONAL USES: Traditionally, He Shou Wu has been used to nourish the liver and kidneys, increase vitality, and to treat issues like thinning hair, premature aging, and high cholesterol. It is often consumed as a tonic in the form of teas, tinctures, and powders.

5. SCIENTIFIC BENEFITS: He Shou Wu is rich in antioxidants and compounds that may help protect the liver, improve kidney function, and boost immune health. It has been shown to have effects on increasing longevity, enhancing blood circulation, and supporting hair growth and color restoration.

6. METAPHYSICAL USES: In metaphysical practices, He Shou Wu is used for its properties of longevity and rejuvenation. It is considered to help in clearing energetic blockages in the body and enhancing spiritual awareness. Practitioners use it in rituals aimed at healing, protection, and personal transformation.

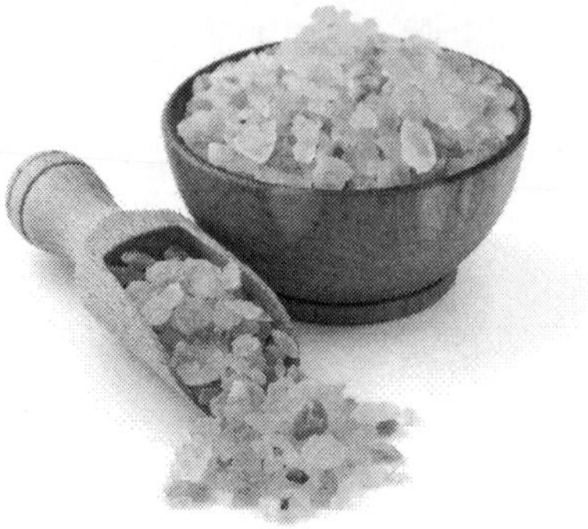

HIMALAYAN SEA SALT

more accurately known as Himalayan Pink Salt, is rock salt mined from the Punjab region of Pakistan, near the foothills of the Himalayas. It is famous for its distinctive pink color, which is due to mineral impurities.

1. DESCRIPTION: Himalayan Pink Salt typically appears in crystal form ranging from off-white to deep pink and even red, depending on the mineral concentration. It is manually extracted and minimally processed to yield an unrefined product rich in minerals.

2. LOCATION: The main source of Himalayan Pink Salt is the Khewra Salt Mine in Pakistan, which is one of the oldest and largest salt mines in the world.

3. GROWING CONDITIONS: Himalayan Pink Salt is a mineral harvested from ancient sea salt deposits that have been compressed over millions of years.

4. TRADITIONAL USES: Historically, Himalayan Pink Salt has been used as a natural preservative and seasoning. Its culinary uses are similar to table salt, including seasoning food, curing meats, and preserving fish.

5. SCIENTIFIC BENEFITS: Himalayan Pink Salt contains over 80 minerals and trace elements, including potassium, iron, and calcium, which can help maintain electrolyte balance, improve hydration, and potentially support proper metabolism. It's also touted for its lower sodium content compared to regular table salt.

6. METAPHYSICAL USES: In metaphysical practices, Himalayan Pink Salt is often used for purification and protection. It is used in energy cleansing rituals to dispel negativity, often placed in bowls around the home or used in baths to cleanse the aura.

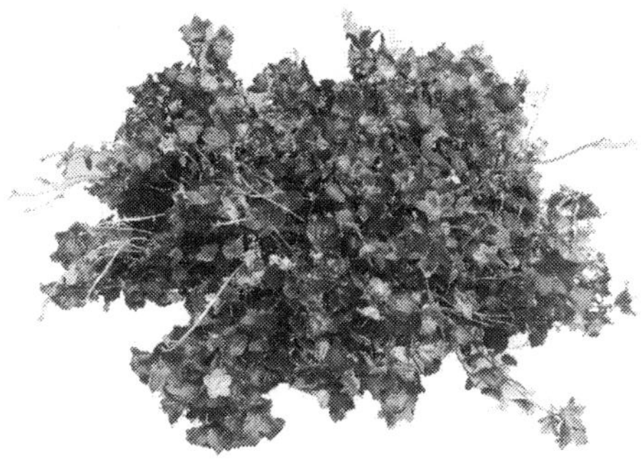

JAMAICAN BLUE VERVAIN

(STACHYTARPHETA JAMAICENSIS)

is a flowering plant native to Jamaica and other parts of the Caribbean. It is recognized for its slender spikes of vibrant blue flowers and its use in traditional medicine.

JAMAICAN BLUE VERVAIN

JAMAICAN BLUE VERVAIN – TINCTURE

1. DESCRIPTION: Jamaican Blue Vervain has elongated, spiky inflorescences of small blue flowers. The plant itself is a perennial with woody stems, small, oblong leaves, and a sprawling growth habit.

2. LOCATION: Native to Jamaica, this herb is also found throughout the Caribbean and has been naturalized in other tropical regions around the world.

3. GROWING CONDITIONS: Jamaican Blue Vervain thrives in well-drained soil, under full sun to partial shade. It prefers tropical climates and is quite drought-resistant once established.

4. TRADITIONAL USES: Traditionally, Jamaican Blue Vervain has been used in herbal medicine to alleviate nervous conditions, insomnia, depression, and even to help with colds and flu. It is also used as a diuretic and for its anti-inflammatory properties.

5. SCIENTIFIC BENEFITS: While scientific research on Jamaican Blue Vervain is limited, the plant is known to contain flavonoids and other compounds that may have anti-inflammatory, analgesic, and sedative effects. It is also valued for its potential to support liver and kidney health.

6. METAPHYSICAL USES: In metaphysical practices, Jamaican Blue Vervain is used for protection and tranquility. It is often used in rituals to promote peace, purify spaces, and attract positive energies. It is believed to help open the mind for spiritual connections and enhance psychic abilities.

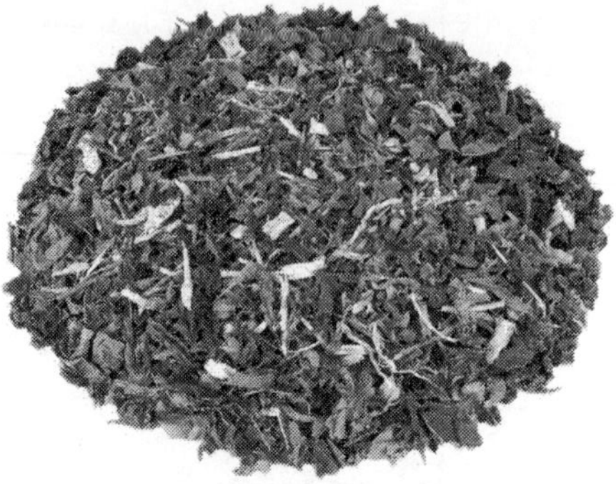

JAMAICAN GUINEA HEN

(PETIVERIA ALLIACEA)

also known as guinea hen weed, anamu, or gully root, is a herbaceous plant native to the Amazon rainforest and the tropical areas of the Caribbean, Central and South America.

1. DESCRIPTION: The plant is recognized for its strong garlic-like odor. It has small greenish-white flowers and grows as a shrub up to about 1 meter tall. The leaves are simple, alternate, and have a slightly wrinkled appearance.

2. LOCATION: While it is native to the tropical parts of the Americas, it is particularly common in Jamaica, where it is widely used in traditional medicine.

3. GROWING CONDITIONS: Jamaican Guinea Hen thrives in warm, humid climates. It prefers well-drained soils and can be found in a variety of environments from shaded areas to open fields.

4. TRADITIONAL USES: Traditionally, it has been used in folk medicine for its anti-inflammatory, analgesic, and antipyretic properties. It is commonly used to treat colds, flu, arthritis, and to boost the immune system. In Jamaica, it is also used as a natural remedy for a wide range of ailments including diabetes and as a general health tonic.

5. SCIENTIFIC BENEFITS: Scientific studies on Jamaican Guinea Hen have shown that it contains compounds with potential anti-cancer properties, especially against prostate and breast cancer cells. It also has antimicrobial, antifungal, and antiviral activities, which make it a potent natural remedy in fighting infections.

6. METAPHYSICAL USES: In metaphysical practices, Jamaican Guinea Hen is used for spiritual cleansing and protection. It is believed to ward off evil spirits and to clear negative energies from a space. It is often used in baths and incense for purification purposes.

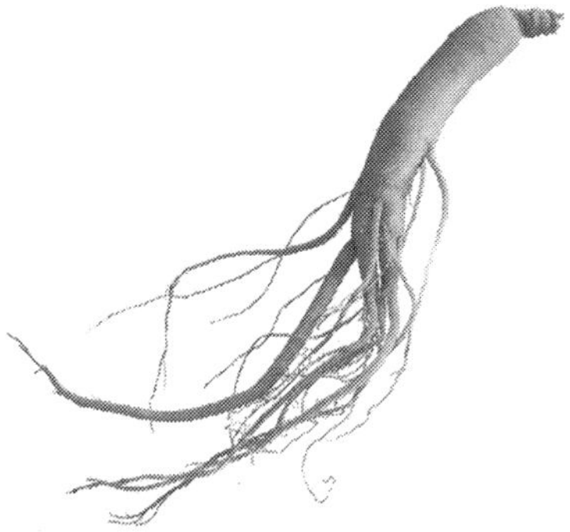

KOREAN GINSENG

(PANAX GINSENG)

also known as Asian or Korean red ginseng, is a perennial plant native to the Korean Peninsula, northeastern China, and far eastern Russia. It is highly prized for its medicinal properties.

1. DESCRIPTION: Korean Ginseng has a distinctive human-like shape for its root, which is thick and fleshy. It has dark green leaves, grouped in a circle, and red berry clusters. The root itself is the most valuable part and can vary in color from pale yellow to red.

2. LOCATION: It is primarily grown in Korea, with significant cultivation also occurring in China and Russia.

3. GROWING CONDITIONS: Korean Ginseng requires a cool climate and well-drained, shaded areas. It is typically grown under forest canopies or in artificially shaded environments. The soil must be rich in organic matter and slightly acidic.

4. TRADITIONAL USES: Traditionally used in East Asian medicine for thousands of years, it is considered a panacea for enhancing longevity and vitality. It is thought to restore and enhance well-being, improve stamina and concentration, and help regulate blood pressure and blood sugar levels.

5. SCIENTIFIC BENEFITS: Korean Ginseng is renowned for its ability to boost the immune system, enhance brain function, fight fatigue, and improve symptoms of erectile dysfunction. It contains several active compounds like ginsenosides and gintonin, which are believed to be responsible for its anti-inflammatory, antioxidant, and neuroprotective effects.

6. METAPHYSICAL USES: In metaphysical practices, Korean Ginseng is used for its properties of vitality and protection. It is believed to enhance personal energy and strength, ward off evil, and attract health and prosperity. It is often used in rituals to increase mental and spiritual power.

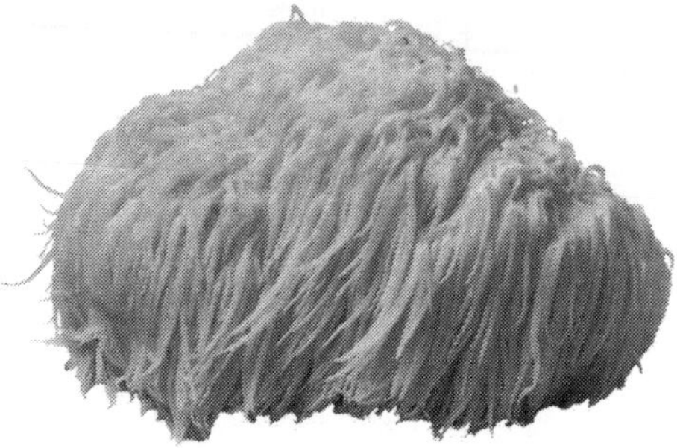

LION'S MANE MUSHROOM

(HERICIUM ERINACEUS)

is a type of edible and medicinal mushroom that grows on hardwood trees. It is known for its unique appearance, resembling a white, shaggy mane of a lion.

1. DESCRIPTION: Lion's Mane has long, flowing, white spines that hang like icicles or a lion's mane, which is how it gets its name. As the mushroom ages, the color can change from pure white to yellowish.

2. LOCATION: This mushroom is found in North America, Europe, and Asia, particularly in temperate forests.

3. GROWING CONDITIONS: Lion's Mane grows best on hardwood trees, such as oaks and beeches. It prefers moist, shaded environments that provide the high humidity necessary for its development.

4. TRADITIONAL USES: Traditionally, Lion's Mane has been used in Chinese and Japanese medicine for its cognitive and neurological health benefits. It is consumed as a gourmet food and used medicinally in tea or supplement form.

5. SCIENTIFIC BENEFITS: Research suggests that Lion's Mane contains bioactive substances that have beneficial effects on the brain, heart, and gut. Studies have shown it may improve cognitive function, reduce symptoms of anxiety and depression, and help repair nerve damage. It also has anti-inflammatory, antioxidant, and immune-boosting properties.

6. METAPHYSICAL USES: In metaphysical practices, Lion's Mane is used for mental clarity and focus. It is believed to enhance spiritual vision and insight, making it a popular choice for meditation and other spiritual activities where mental clarity is sought.

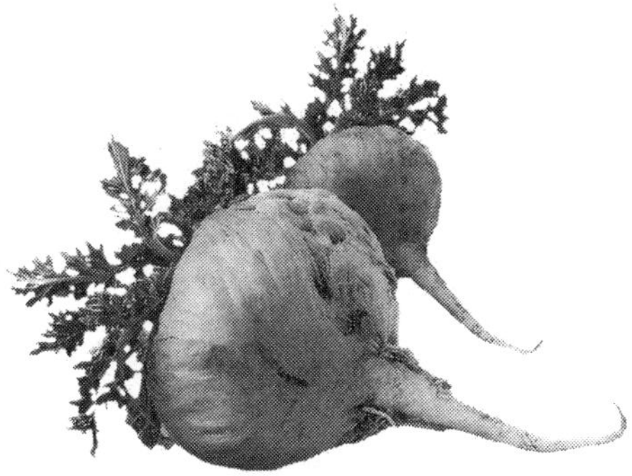

MACA ROOT

(LEPIDIUM MEYENII)

is a cruciferous vegetable native to the high Andes of Peru, often grown at altitudes over 4,000 meters. It is known for its nutritional benefits and as an adaptogen—a substance that helps the body adapt to stress.

MACA ROOT RED

MACA ROOT BLACK

1. DESCRIPTION: Maca root resembles a cross between a radish and a turnip with a rough skin that can range from yellow to purple and black. The root is usually dried and powdered after harvest.

2. LOCATION: Maca is primarily grown in the central Andes of Peru, in harsh conditions and at very high altitudes where few other plants can survive.

3. GROWING CONDITIONS: Maca thrives in cold, high altitude climates with poor, rocky soil. It is a hardy plant that requires minimal water and resists strong winds and sunlight.

4. TRADITIONAL USES: Traditionally, maca has been used as a food source and in medicine. The Incas consumed it for its energy and stamina-enhancing properties, and it has been used to improve sexual health, reproductive health, and hormone balance.

5. SCIENTIFIC BENEFITS: Maca is rich in vitamins, minerals, essential amino acids, and phytonutrients, making it a powerful nutrient booster. It is known for increasing libido, reducing erectile dysfunction, boosting energy and endurance, improving mood, and potentially reducing blood pressure and sun damage. Studies also suggest that it can help improve memory and learning.

6. METAPHYSICAL USES: In metaphysical practices, maca is often used for its energizing and revitalizing properties. It is believed to increase strength, stamina, and to balance the body's energetic fields. Maca is used in rituals aimed at boosting vitality and resilience.

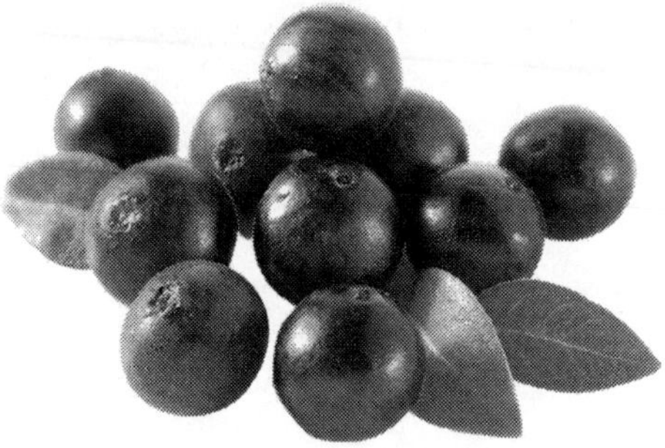

MAQUI BERRIES

(ARISTOTELIA CHILENSIS)

are small, dark purple berries native to the rainforests of Chile and Argentina. They are highly prized for their antioxidant properties and are considered a superfood.

1. DESCRIPTION: Maqui berries are small, round, and have a deep purple to almost black color, indicative of their high anthocyanin content. They are similar in size to blueberries but have a slightly tart, sweet flavor.

2. LOCATION: Primarily found in the temperate rainforests of southern Chile and parts of western Argentina.

3. GROWING CONDITIONS: Maqui berries grow on small trees or large shrubs in the dense understorey of the South American rainforest. They thrive in well-drained soils, in areas with high rainfall and cool temperatures.

4. TRADITIONAL USES: Historically, the Mapuche Indians have consumed maqui berries for their medicinal properties, using them to treat inflammation, diarrhea, and ulcers, and as a general tonic to improve stamina and strength.

5. SCIENTIFIC BENEFITS: Maqui berries are exceptionally rich in antioxidants, particularly anthocyanins, which may help combat oxidative stress and reduce inflammation. Research suggests they have potential benefits for regulating blood sugar levels, improving cardiovascular health, and aiding in weight management. Their antioxidant properties may also support eye health and skin vitality.

6. METAPHYSICAL USES: In metaphysical practices, maqui berries are used for purification and protection. They are believed to cleanse the body and spirit of toxins and negative energies, enhancing overall vitality and protection.

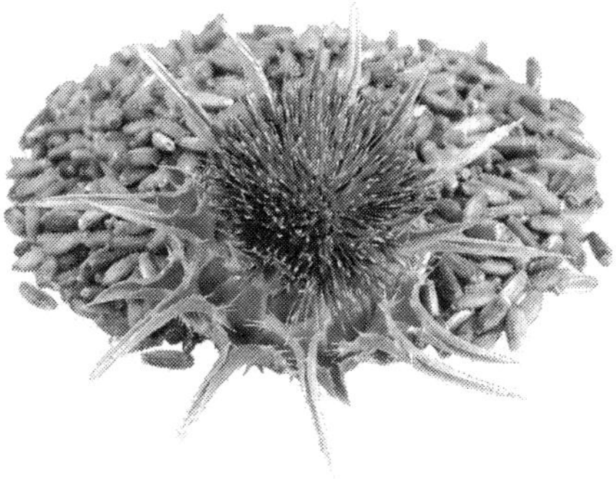

MILK THISTLE

(SILYBUM MARIANUM)

is a flowering plant native to Mediterranean countries. It's known for its distinctive purple flowers and white-veined leaves, and it has been used medicinally for over 2,000 years.

1. DESCRIPTION: Milk thistle plants can grow to be quite tall, up to 10 feet, with spiky leaves and a large, purple to pink thistle at the top. The leaves are glossy green with white veins, which give them a marbled appearance.

2. LOCATION: Originally from the Mediterranean, milk thistle is now found throughout the world, including North America and Australia. It typically grows in dry, rocky soils.

3. GROWING CONDITIONS: Milk thistle prefers sunny conditions and well-drained soils but is quite tolerant of poor soil conditions. It is often found in waste areas and along roadsides.

4. TRADITIONAL USES: Traditionally, milk thistle has been used to treat liver and gallbladder disorders. The seeds are the most commonly used part of the plant, used to make extracts or teas.

5. SCIENTIFIC BENEFITS: Milk thistle is best known for its liver-protecting effects. It contains silymarin, a group of compounds said to have antioxidant and anti-inflammatory properties. Silymarin has been studied for its potential to support liver health by promoting liver cell regeneration, protecting against liver damage from toxins, and helping manage liver diseases such as cirrhosis and hepatitis.

6. METAPHYSICAL USES: In metaphysical practices, milk thistle is used for protection, especially against poisonous thoughts and emotions. It is believed to provide protective energy that wards off negativity and evil, making it useful in spells and potions intended to shield and cleanse.

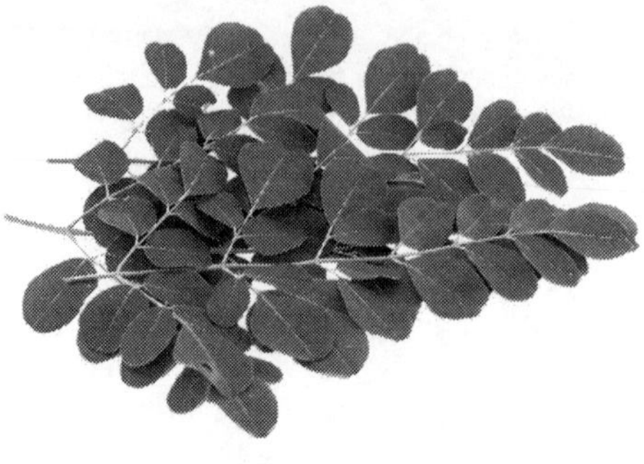

MORINGA

(MORINGA OLEIFERA)

often called the drumstick tree, miracle tree, or horseradish tree, is a fast-growing, drought-resistant tree native to the Indian subcontinent. It is highly valued for its nutritional content and various medicinal benefits.

MORINGA POWDER

MORINGA SEEDS

1. DESCRIPTION: Moringa trees can reach up to 10-12 meters in height. They have fragile branches, delicate leaves, and long, pod-like fruits called drumsticks. Both the leaves and seeds of the Moringa tree are used for their health benefits.

2. LOCATION: While native to parts of India, Pakistan, Bangladesh, and Afghanistan, Moringa is now cultivated in many tropical and subtropical areas around the world, including Africa and South America.

3. GROWING CONDITIONS: Moringa thrives in warm, sunny environments and is highly tolerant of drought and poor soil, although it prefers well-drained sandy or loamy soil.

4. TRADITIONAL USES: Traditionally, Moringa leaves have been used in cooking and medicine in many cultures. They are rich in nutrients and antioxidants, and are used to combat malnutrition, especially among infants and nursing mothers. The seeds are used for their oil, to purify water and its traditional uses of maintaining healthy cholesterol and blood sugar levels .

5. SCIENTIFIC BENEFITS: Moringa leaves are exceptionally nutritious, rich in vitamins A, C, and E, calcium, potassium, and protein. They have been shown to reduce blood sugar levels, improve heart health by reducing cholesterol, and possess anti-inflammatory and antioxidant properties. Moringa seeds also have antifungal, antiviral, antidepressant, and anti-inflammatory properties.

6. METAPHYSICAL USES: In metaphysical practices, Moringa is used for protection and nourishment. It is believed to bring health and vitality when used in spells and rituals, and to provide spiritual nourishment, as it does physically.

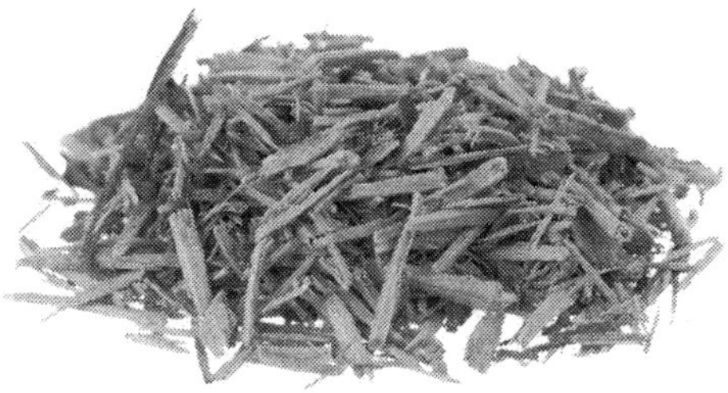

MUIRA PUAMA

(PTYCHOPETALUM OLACOIDES)

also known as "potency wood," is a bush native to the Brazilian Amazon. It is renowned for its use in the traditional medicine of the region, particularly as an aphrodisiac and stimulant.

1. DESCRIPTION: Muira Puama is a small tree or shrub that grows about 14 feet high. It has small white flowers and produces small, dark fruits. The roots and bark of the tree are the parts most commonly used for their medicinal properties.

2. LOCATION: It is found primarily in the Amazon rainforest, particularly in Brazil, but also in parts of Peru and Guyana.

3. GROWING CONDITIONS: Muira Puama grows in the rich soil of the Amazon rainforest. It thrives in tropical, humid conditions and requires a moderate amount of shade.

4. TRADITIONAL USES: Traditionally, Muira Puama has been used by indigenous cultures in the Amazon for treating a variety of ailments, including sexual dysfunction, nerve pain, digestive problems, and as a general tonic to boost energy and mental focus.

5. SCIENTIFIC BENEFITS: While research is limited, Muira Puama is often used to increase libido and sexual function. Studies suggest it may help with relaxation of the corpus cavernosa — one of the chambers of the penis — potentially improving erectile function. It is also noted for its adaptogenic and neuroprotective potential, which may aid in combating stress and improving cognitive function.

6. METAPHYSICAL USES: In metaphysical practices, Muira Puama is used for its energizing and grounding properties. It is believed to enhance physical strength and endurance, as well as to increase personal power and protect against negative energies.

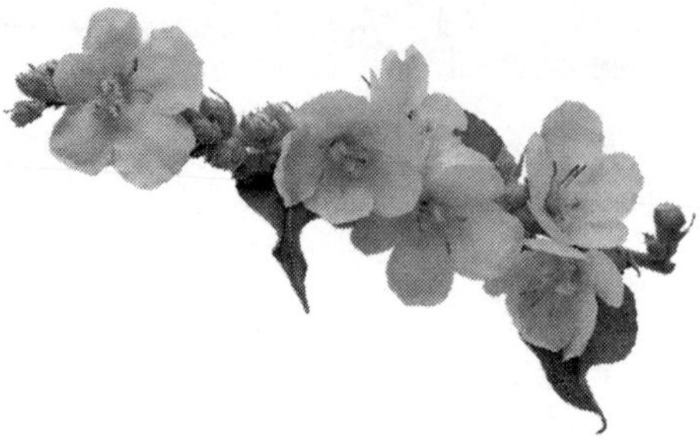

MULLEIN

(VERBASCUM THAPSUS)

also known as great mullein or common mullein, is a biennial herb known for its tall, dense spikes of yellow flowers and soft, velvety leaves.

1. DESCRIPTION: Mullein plants can grow up to 2 meters tall, featuring a rosette of large, woolly, oblong leaves in the first year and a tall, rod-like stem with dense clusters of yellow flowers in the second year. The leaves and flowers are both used medicinally.

2. LOCATION: Originally native to Europe, Asia, and North Africa, mullein has been naturalized across North America and Australia. It's commonly found in fields, meadows, and waste areas where the soil is well-drained and sandy.

3. GROWING CONDITIONS: Mullein prefers full sun and well-drained soil. It is drought-resistant and often grows in poor soil, making it a common plant in disturbed areas.

4. TRADITIONAL USES: Historically, mullein has been used for its effectiveness in treating respiratory conditions. It has been used in traditional medicine as a remedy for bronchitis, asthma, pneumonia, and coughs. The leaves are often used to make teas, tinctures, or smoked to relieve chest congestion.

5. SCIENTIFIC BENEFITS: The flowers and leaves of mullein contain saponins, mucilage, and flavonoids, which contribute to its soothing, anti-inflammatory, and antispasmodic properties. It is particularly valued for its ability to relieve irritation of the mucous membranes, helping to clear congestion from the lungs.

6. METAPHYSICAL USES: In metaphysical practices, mullein is often used for protection and cleansing. It is believed to ward off evil and negativity, often used in spells or carried as a charm. Mullein is also used in rituals to instill courage and provide health protection.

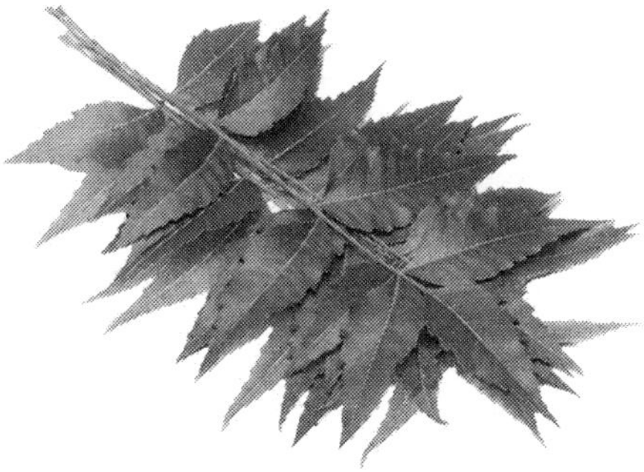

NEEM LEAF

comes from the Neem tree (Azadirachta indica), a tree native to the Indian subcontinent. It is valued for its medicinal properties and is a staple in Ayurvedic medicine.

1. DESCRIPTION: Neem leaves are green, pinnate (divided like a feather), with serrated edges. They are typically 20-40 cm long, with 20 to 31 medium to dark green leaflets about 3 to 8 cm long.

2. LOCATION: Originally from India, neem trees are now found in many parts of Asia, Africa, and the Americas in similar tropical and subtropical climates.

3. GROWING CONDITIONS: Neem trees thrive in areas with sub-arid to sub-humid conditions, with annual rainfall of 400-1,200 mm. They are highly adaptable to a wide range of soils but grow best on well-drained deep and sandy soils.

4. TRADITIONAL USES: Traditionally, neem leaves are used to treat a variety of ailments including ulcers, fever, leprosy, and malaria. They are also used in dental and skin care products for their antiseptic properties.

5. SCIENTIFIC BENEFITS: Neem leaves are rich in compounds with antifungal, antibacterial, and anti-inflammatory properties. They are used for treating skin conditions like acne and eczema, for dental care in toothpastes and mouthwashes, and even as an insect repellent.

6. METAPHYSICAL USES: In metaphysical practices, neem is often used for protection. It is believed to cleanse the aura, purify spaces, and protect against negative energies. Neem leaves are sometimes kept in homes to ward off evil spirits.

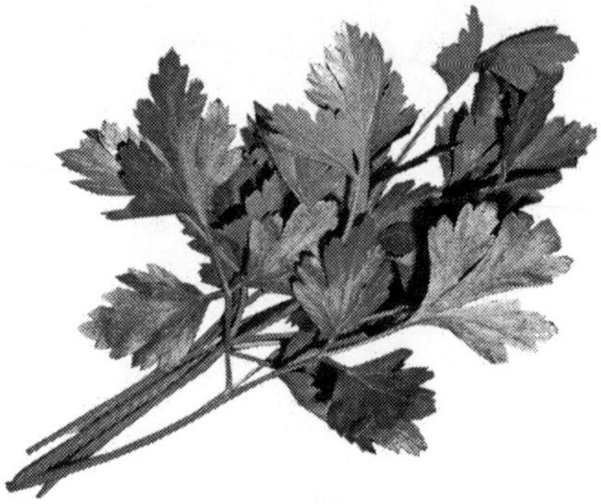

PARSLEY

(PETROSELINUM CRISPUM)

is a widely used culinary and medicinal herb native to the central Mediterranean region (southern Italy, Greece, Portugal, Spain, Malta, Morocco, and Tunisia).

1. DESCRIPTION: Parsley is a bright green, biennial plant in temperate climates, although it is often cultivated as an annual. It features curly or flat leaves, depending on the variety, which are finely divided and sprout from a central point.

2. LOCATION: While native to the Mediterranean, parsley is now cultivated worldwide for culinary use and can thrive in most temperate climates.

3. GROWING CONDITIONS: Parsley grows best in moist, well-drained soil, under full sun to partial shade. It prefers cooler temperatures and may bolt (flower and go to seed) in peak summer heat.

4. TRADITIONAL USES: Parsley is extensively used as a garnish, a flavor enhancer in cooking, and in herbal medicine, it has been used to treat conditions like high blood pressure and allergies. It's also a common component in green smoothies and juices for its nutritional benefits.

5. SCIENTIFIC BENEFITS: Parsley is rich in vitamins A, C, and K, and has antioxidant properties. It supports bone health, enhances immune function, and its high vitamin K content helps with blood clotting. Parsley also contains myristicin, a natural compound thought to support liver health and detoxification.

6. METAPHYSICAL USES: In metaphysical practices, parsley is used to promote love and protection. It is often used in rituals to clear out negative energies and bring about personal purification. Parsley is also associated with death and rebirth, featuring in rituals that involve endings and new beginnings.

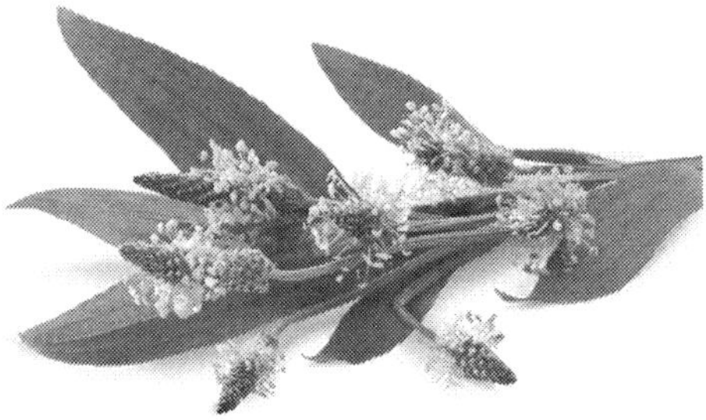

PLANTAIN

(often referred to as common plantain, Plantago major) is a herbaceous perennial plant native to Europe and Asia but now found worldwide. It is distinct from the banana-like fruit also called plantain.

1. DESCRIPTION: Plantain has a rosette of dark green, oval to oblong leaves that grow close to the ground. The leaves are smooth and have prominent parallel veins. It produces a flower spike that is greenish-brown, with tiny, densely packed flowers.

2. LOCATION: While native to Europe and parts of Asia, common plantain has become naturalized across the globe, including North America, Australia, and other parts of Asia. It often grows in compacted soils along paths, roadsides, and in lawns.

3. GROWING CONDITIONS: Plantain prefers compacted, poor soils and is highly adaptable to different environmental conditions. It thrives in full sun to partial shade.

4. TRADITIONAL USES: Traditionally, plantain has been used for its medicinal properties. It is known for its ability to treat skin conditions, such as wounds and insect bites, due to its anti-inflammatory and antibacterial properties. The leaves are often used in poultices or infused as a tea to treat respiratory issues or digestive problems.

5. SCIENTIFIC BENEFITS: Plantain leaves contain allantoin, an anti-inflammatory compound that promotes wound healing, stimulates the growth of new skin cells, and soothes inflamed skin. It is also a good source of vitamins C and K, and dietary fiber.

6. METAPHYSICAL USES: In metaphysical practices, plantain is used for healing, protection, and strength. It is believed to ward off snakes and other venomous creatures, both physically and spiritually. Plantain is often used in spells to promote healing and to protect against negativity.

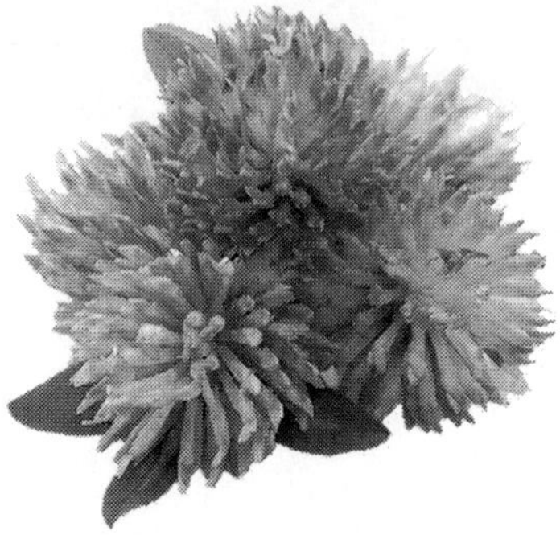

RED CLOVER

(TRIFOLIUM PRATENSE)

is a perennial herbaceous plant native to Europe, Western Asia, and northwest Africa. It has since been naturalized in many other regions as a pasture crop.

1. DESCRIPTION: Red clover has trifoliate (three-part) leaves and distinctive round, pink to red flowers. The plant is relatively short, growing only about 20-80 cm tall, with hairy stems and leaves.

2. LOCATION: While originally from Europe and parts of Asia, red clover is now widespread across North America and Australia, primarily used in agriculture as fodder and a soil improver.

3. GROWING CONDITIONS: Red clover prefers well-drained soils rich in calcium but can adapt to a variety of soil types. It thrives in full sunlight and requires moderate amounts of water.

4. TRADITIONAL USES: Traditionally, red clover flowers have been used in herbal medicine to treat a variety of conditions including skin disorders, asthma, and as a detoxifying herb. It is also used as an expectorant and for menopausal symptoms due to its isoflavone content.

5. SCIENTIFIC BENEFITS: Red clover is rich in isoflavones, which are plant-based chemicals that act like estrogen in the body. This makes it particularly beneficial for alleviating menopause symptoms such as hot flashes and bone density loss. It also has anti-inflammatory properties and supports cardiovascular health by improving arterial flexibility and reducing cholesterol levels.

6. METAPHYSICAL USES: In metaphysical practices, red clover is often used for protection and prosperity. It is believed to ward off negative spirits and is used in potions and spells to promote financial success, as well as to enhance fidelity and commitment in relationships.

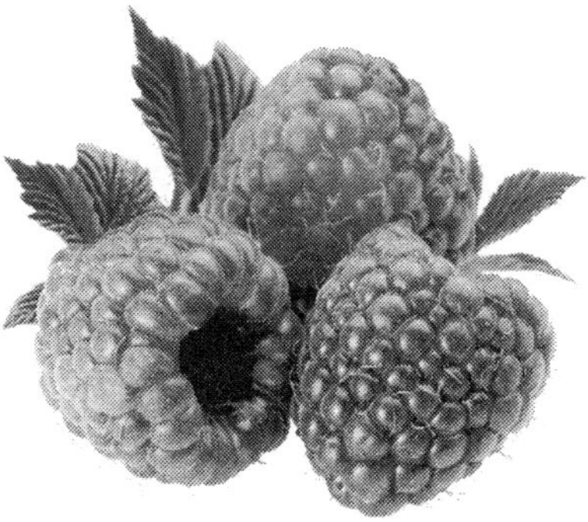

RED RASPBERRY LEAF

(RUBUS IDAEUS)

is part of the raspberry plant, known for its delicious fruit. The leaves of the raspberry plant have been used traditionally in herbal medicine, especially concerning women's health.

1. DESCRIPTION: Red raspberry leaves are green, pinnate, and have a rough texture with a silvery underside. They resemble the shape of a maple leaf but are smaller and more delicate.

2. LOCATION: Native to Europe and parts of Asia, red raspberry has been widely cultivated in many temperate regions around the world, including North America.

3. GROWING CONDITIONS: Red raspberry plants prefer cool climates with well-drained, fertile soil. They thrive in full sun to partial shade and require regular watering during the growing season.

4. TRADITIONAL USES: The leaves have been used traditionally as a herbal remedy for various ailments, particularly for women. They are most commonly used to tone the uterus, reduce menstrual cramps, and manage labor pains during childbirth.

5. SCIENTIFIC BENEFITS: Red raspberry leaves are rich in vitamins and minerals including vitamins C, E, and B complex, as well as magnesium, potassium, and iron. They contain tannins that are thought to strengthen the uterine muscles and improve labor outcomes. The leaves are also believed to have anti-inflammatory and antioxidant properties.

6. METAPHYSICAL USES: In metaphysical practices, red raspberry leaf is used for protection and to promote fertility and feminine health. It is often used in spells and rituals related to female empowerment, motherhood, and pregnancy.

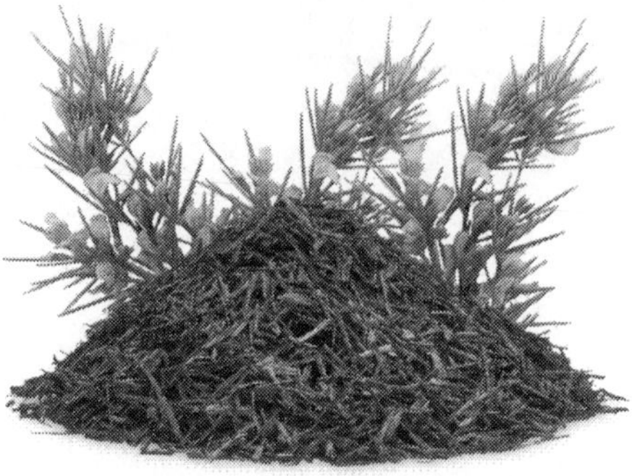

RED ROOIBOS TEA

comes from the plant Aspalathus linearis, which is native to the Cederberg region of South Africa. It is not a true tea but a herbaceous plant that produces leaves used to make an herbal tea known for its unique flavor and health benefits.

1. DESCRIPTION: Red Rooibos has needle-like leaves that are green when fresh but turn red upon fermentation. The plant itself is a leguminous shrub that grows about 1-2 meters tall.

2. LOCATION: Rooibos is exclusively grown in the Cederberg mountains of the Western Cape province of South Africa, a region with unique soil and climatic conditions ideal for its growth.

3. GROWING CONDITIONS: Rooibos thrives in the Cederberg's sandy soil and requires hot and dry summer conditions to grow. It is drought-resistant and adapted to survive the harsh conditions of its native environment.

4. TRADITIONAL USES: Traditionally, rooibos tea has been consumed for its potential health benefits, including soothing stomach cramps, aiding digestion, and providing relief from allergies and asthma. It's a staple drink in South Africa and is gaining popularity worldwide.

5. SCIENTIFIC BENEFITS: Rooibos tea is caffeine-free, low in tannins, and rich in antioxidants such as aspalathin and nothofagin, which are rare in other plants. These antioxidants help protect against cell damage caused by free radicals. Studies suggest that rooibos may also benefit heart health by improving cholesterol levels and blood pressure.

6. METAPHYSICAL USES: In metaphysical practices, red rooibos tea is often used for calming and grounding effects. It is believed to support emotional balance and help with clearing away old, stagnant energies. It's used in rituals focused on healing, peace, and tranquility.

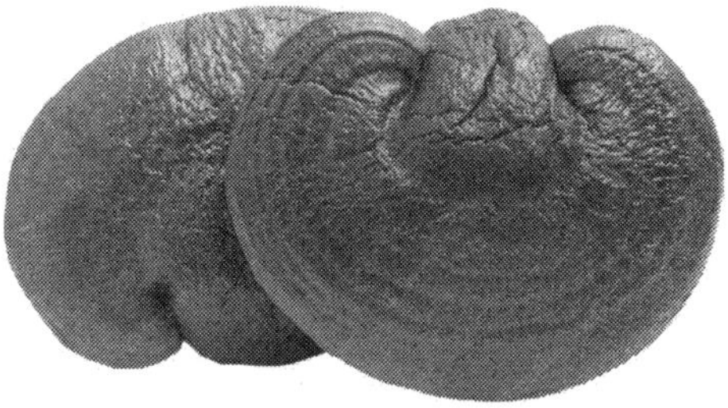

REISHI MUSHROOM

(GANODERMA LUCIDUM)

also known as Lingzhi, is a fungus celebrated for its medicinal properties. It is native to several regions of Asia and is a staple in traditional Eastern medicine.

1. DESCRIPTION: Reishi mushrooms have a distinctive appearance with a shiny, varnished, reddish-brown cap that is kidney-shaped and flat. They grow on hardwoods and are often found on logs and trees in forested areas.

2. LOCATION: Native to humid, coastal regions of China and Japan, Reishi is now cultivated worldwide in both controlled and natural environments due to its valued properties.

3. GROWING CONDITIONS: Reishi grows naturally on hardwoods like maples and oaks. For cultivation, it requires high humidity and temperatures between 24-30°C. It grows slowly, taking several months to develop fully.

4. TRADITIONAL USES: Traditionally, Reishi has been used to support immune function, reduce stress, and promote longevity and health. It is considered the "mushroom of immortality" in traditional Chinese medicine and is used to treat a wide range of diseases and conditions.

5. SCIENTIFIC BENEFITS: Reishi mushrooms are rich in polysaccharides, triterpenoids, and peptidoglycans, which contribute to their health-promoting properties. Studies suggest that Reishi can enhance immune response, reduce inflammation, and help fight fatigue and depression. It also supports cardiovascular health and may help in managing blood pressure and cholesterol levels.

6. METAPHYSICAL USES: In metaphysical practices, Reishi is used for its spiritual and protective benefits. It is believed to protect against negative energy and to enhance spiritual connection and wisdom. Reishi is often used in practices aimed at meditation and spiritual growth.

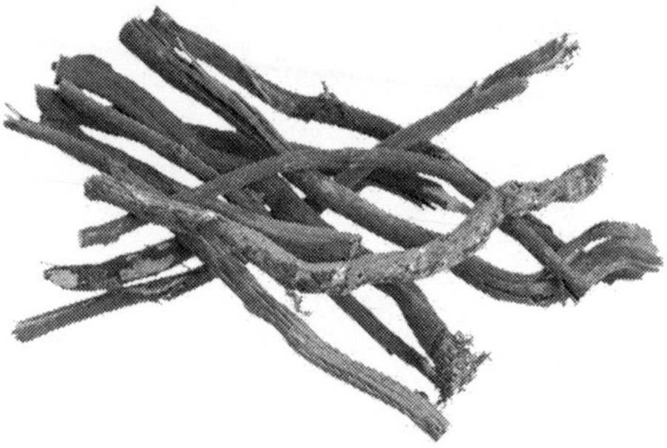

SARSAPARILLA ROOT

comes from several species of the genus Smilax, but the most commonly used for medicinal purposes are Smilax ornata and Smilax regelii. It is native to South America, Jamaica, the Caribbean, Mexico, and Honduras.

1. DESCRIPTION: Sarsaparilla plants are climbing, woody vines that grow long, thin roots. The roots are often brown or gray, have a fragrant aroma, and a slightly spicy taste.

2. LOCATION: Originally from the tropical regions of the Americas, Sarsaparilla is now also cultivated in parts of Asia, especially in India and China, for its medicinal uses.

3. GROWING CONDITIONS: Sarsaparilla thrives in warm, moist environments. It grows best in rich, well-drained soil with partial shade, as direct sunlight can be too intense.

4. TRADITIONAL USES: Traditionally, Sarsaparilla root has been used for its detoxifying properties. It was popularly used in traditional medicine to treat skin diseases, rheumatism, and sexually transmitted diseases like syphilis. It was also used as the primary flavoring in traditional root beer.

5. SCIENTIFIC BENEFITS: Sarsaparilla contains compounds such as saponins, flavonoids, and plant sterols, which have anti-inflammatory and antioxidant properties. These compounds may help treat skin conditions like psoriasis, eczema, and acne. There is also evidence suggesting that Sarsaparilla can bind to endotoxins in the gut, aiding in their removal from the body.

6. METAPHYSICAL USES: In metaphysical practices, Sarsaparilla is used for purification and protection. It is believed to have the ability to cleanse the blood and, by extension, clear negative energies from the body. Sarsaparilla is used in rituals aimed at physical and spiritual detoxification.

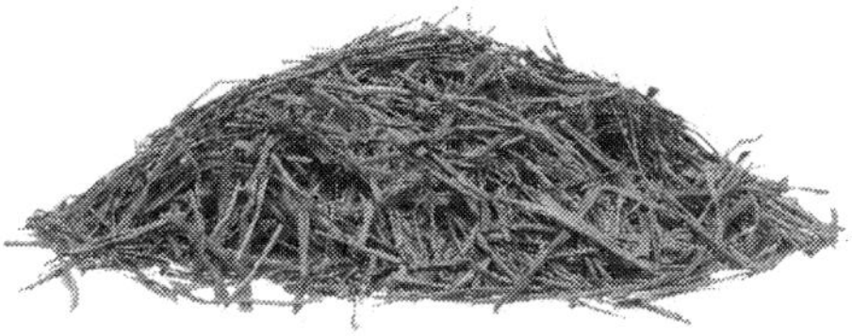

SENCHA GREEN TEA

is a type of Japanese green tea, made from the leaves of the Camellia sinensis plant. It is the most popular tea in Japan, celebrated for its delicate balance of sweetness and astringency.

1. DESCRIPTION: Sencha leaves are initially steamed, rolled, and then dried, forming slender, needle-like shapes. The tea itself has a bright green color when brewed and offers a refreshing, grassy flavor.

2. LOCATION: While Sencha is predominantly produced in Japan, regions known for their high-quality Sencha include Shizuoka, Kagoshima, and Uji.

3. GROWING CONDITIONS: Sencha thrives in regions with a mix of sun and light shade, benefiting from misty climates with rich, volcanic soil that drains well.

4. TRADITIONAL USES: Traditionally, Sencha is consumed daily in Japan, serving both social and ceremonial purposes. It is appreciated not just for its flavor but also for its role in promoting wellness and relaxation.

5. SCIENTIFIC BENEFITS: Sencha is rich in antioxidants, particularly catechins, which have cancer-fighting properties and may help prevent heart disease. The tea is also a good source of vitamin C, contributing to immune system health, skin quality, and stress reduction. Additionally, it contains theanine, an amino acid that can enhance calmness and alertness.

6. METAPHYSICAL USES: In metaphysical practices, Sencha is used to promote clarity, cleansing, and rejuvenation. It is often used in rituals to purify the mind and body, promote healing, and bring about peace and balance.

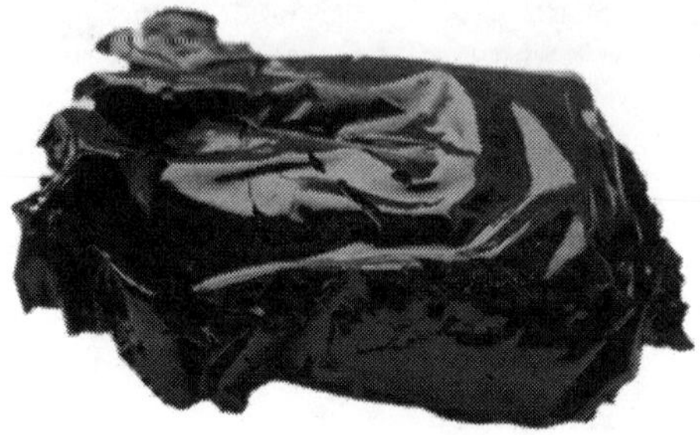

SHILAJIT

is a sticky, tar-like substance found primarily in the rocks of the Himalayas. It develops over centuries from the slow decomposition of plants and is commonly used in Ayurvedic medicine.

SHILAJIT RESIN

SHILAJIT TABLETS

1. DESCRIPTION: Shilajit appears as a thick, dark resin that exudes from cracks in mountain rocks during warm weather. It is composed of humus and organic plant materials that have been compressed by layers of rock.

2. LOCATION: Shilajit is predominantly found in the Himalayan region, including India, Nepal, Bhutan, and also in other mountain ranges such as the Altai, the Caucasus, and the Gilgit-Baltistan region of Pakistan.

3. GROWING CONDITIONS: Shilajit forms in specific geological conditions in high mountain ranges, primarily from the decomposition of certain plants by the action of microorganisms. It is collected from rocks at altitudes between 1,000 to 5,000 meters.

4. TRADITIONAL USES: Traditionally, Shilajit has been praised for its rejuvenating and adaptogenic effects, enhancing physical strength and recovering energy. It's been used to support digestion, improve stamina, and as a natural remedy for many ailments including anemia, arthritis, asthma, and even diabetes.

5. SCIENTIFIC BENEFITS: Shilajit contains fulvic acid, a potent antioxidant and anti-inflammatory compound, which helps in reducing cellular damage and inflammation. It is also rich in minerals and other organic substances that may contribute to its effects on improving stamina and muscular strength, enhancing the rejuvenation of cells, and managing stress levels. Research has indicated potential benefits in controlling cognitive disorders linked to aging.

6. METAPHYSICAL USES: In metaphysical practices, Shilajit is often used to enhance spiritual growth and promote longevity. It is believed to ground and rejuvenate not only the physical body but also to align the spiritual essence within, aiding in the balance of life force energy.

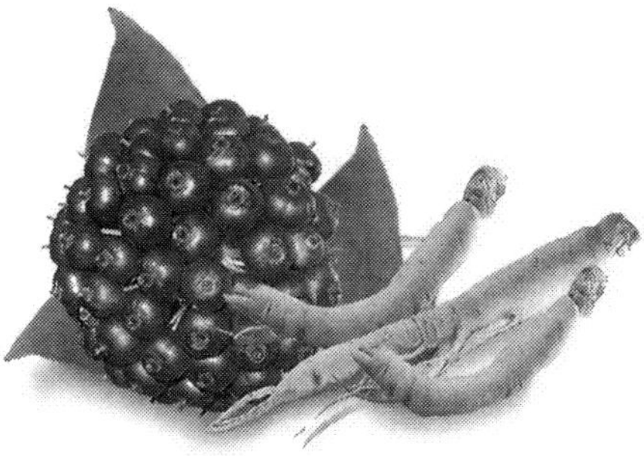

SIBERIAN GINSENG

(ELEUTHEROCOCCUS SENTICOSUS)

also known as Eleuthero, is not a true ginseng but is so named because of its similar properties and uses. It is native to northeastern Asia, including parts of Russia, China, Korea, and Japan.

1. DESCRIPTION: Siberian Ginseng is a small, woody shrub with thorny stems, palmate leaves, and small black berries. It is the root that is primarily used in herbal supplements.

2. LOCATION: It grows in the mountainous regions of Siberia, northern China, Korea, and Japan.

3. GROWING CONDITIONS: This plant thrives in cold climates and can be found in the dense underbrush of the forest. It prefers well-drained soils and tolerates partial shade.

4. TRADITIONAL USES: Traditionally, Siberian Ginseng has been used to increase energy, enhance stamina, reduce fatigue, and minimize stress effects. It has been a staple in traditional Chinese medicine and Russian folk medicine for centuries.

5. SCIENTIFIC BENEFITS: Siberian Ginseng is known as an adaptogen, which helps the body better handle and adapt to stress. It has compounds that may boost the immune system, help fight off colds and flu, increase mental performance, and improve physical stamina. Research also suggests that it can help normalize blood pressure and reduce the severity of heart disease.

6. METAPHYSICAL USES: In metaphysical practices, Siberian Ginseng is used for energy, vitality, and protection. It is believed to enhance personal power and resilience, protect against negative energies, and promote healing and recovery.

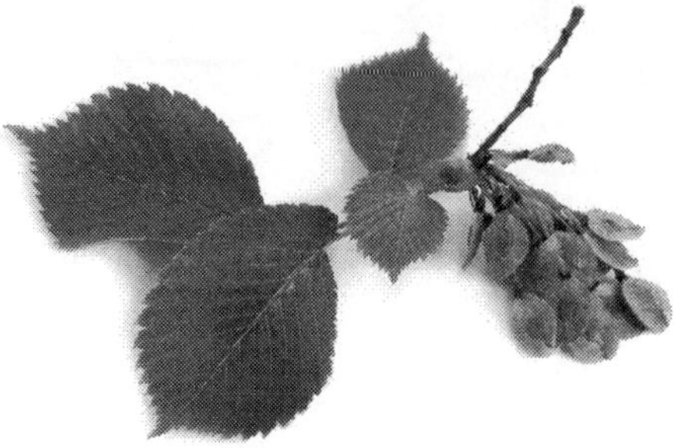

SLIPPERY ELM

(ULMUS RUBRA)

also known as red elm, is a tree native to North America, widely valued for the medicinal properties of its inner bark.

1. DESCRIPTION: Slippery Elm is a medium-sized tree that can reach up to 20 meters in height. Its inner bark is the most utilized part, which becomes slimy or "slippery" when moistened. This mucilage is odorless and has a slightly sweet taste.

2. LOCATION: Native to eastern North America, it ranges from parts of Canada down to the northern parts of Florida and Texas in the United States.

3. GROWING CONDITIONS: Slippery Elm prefers moist, rich soils and part-sun to part-shade conditions. It is commonly found in the deciduous forests of the Eastern and Central United States.

4. TRADITIONAL USES: Traditionally, the inner bark of slippery elm has been used as a remedy for sore throats, coughs, dryness of the lungs, and digestive issues. It is also used externally for healing wounds, burns, and skin inflammation.

5. SCIENTIFIC BENEFITS: The mucilaginous properties of Slippery Elm bark make it effective in soothing the mucous membranes. It can help relieve inflammatory conditions of the gastrointestinal tract, such as gastritis, esophagitis, and irritable bowel syndrome (IBS). Its soothing effect is also beneficial for respiratory ailments and sore throats.

6. METAPHYSICAL USES: In metaphysical practices, Slippery Elm is used for protection and halting gossip. It is believed to shield against slander and to stop lies. It's often used in spells that involve silencing backtalk or protecting against malicious intents.

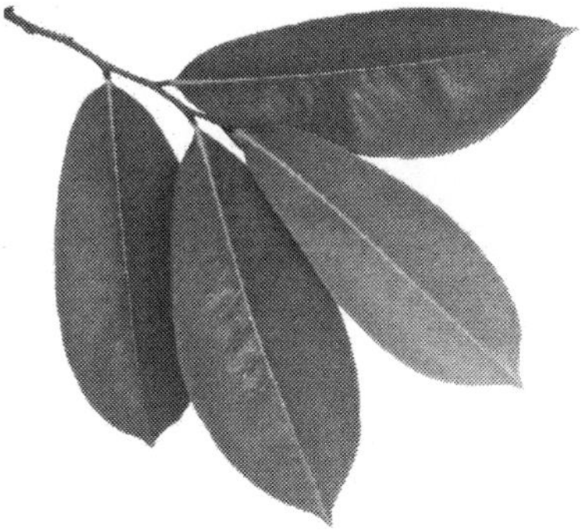

SOURSOP

(ANNONA MURICATA)

also known as graviola or Brazilian paw paw, is a fruit-bearing tree known for its distinctive, spiky green fruit and its medicinal leaves.

SOURSOP POWDER

SOURSOP DRIED LEAVES

1. DESCRIPTION: Soursop trees can grow up to 9 meters tall. The fruit is large, typically weighing 1 to 5 kilograms, with a soft, spiny green exterior and a creamy, fibrous white interior. The taste of soursop is a unique combination of strawberry and pineapple, with a hint of citrus and a creamy texture akin to banana or coconut.

2. LOCATION: Native to the tropical regions of the Americas and the Caribbean, soursop is also cultivated in some parts of Africa, Southeast Asia, and Florida.

3. GROWING CONDITIONS: Soursop thrives in warm, humid climates. It prefers well-drained, sandy loam soils with a pH of 5 to 6.5. The tree requires regular watering and does not tolerate cold temperatures or drought.

4. TRADITIONAL USES: Traditionally, soursop fruit is consumed fresh or used in beverages, smoothies, and desserts. The leaves of the soursop tree are often used in traditional medicine for their purported health benefits. They are commonly brewed into a tea thought to help treat stomach ailments, fever, parasitic infections, hypertension, and rheumatism.

5. SCIENTIFIC BENEFITS: Soursop is rich in vitamins C and B, antioxidants, and a number of phytochemicals. It has been studied for its potential anti-cancer properties, particularly through its content of acetogenins, which may inhibit the growth of cancer cells. The fruit and leaves also have anti-inflammatory, antiviral, and antimicrobial properties. However, more clinical studies are needed to fully establish these health benefits.

6. METAPHYSICAL USES: In metaphysical practices, soursop is used for healing and protection. The leaves and fruit are believed to help cleanse the body and spirit of negative energies, promote healing from illness, and provide protection against spiritual attacks.

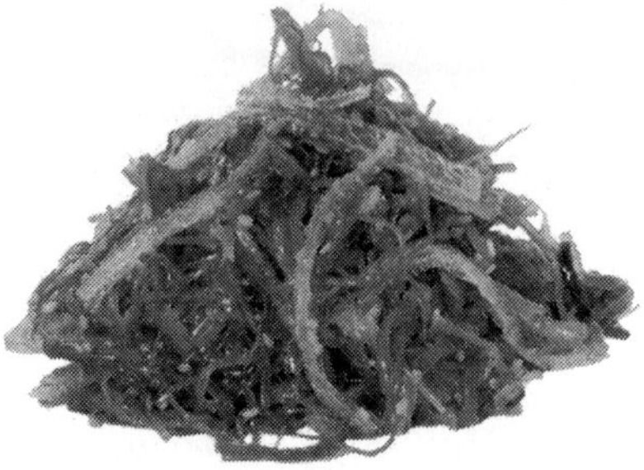

SPIRULINA

is a type of blue-green algae that grows naturally in mineral-rich alkaline lakes. It is renowned for its intense green color and its impressive nutritional profile.

1. DESCRIPTION: Spirulina appears as fine, filamentous, spiral-shaped microalgae. It is often harvested from controlled environments and sold as a dietary supplement in powder, tablet, or capsule form.

2. LOCATION: While naturally found in lakes of Africa, Asia, and South America, spirulina is extensively cultivated in countries like the USA, Thailand, India, and China under controlled conditions to ensure purity and maximize nutrient content.

3. GROWING CONDITIONS: Spirulina thrives in warm, alkaline waters rich in nutrients, particularly carbonates and bicarbonates. It requires a pH of around 8.5–11 and temperatures that range from 30°C to 37°C.

4. TRADITIONAL USES: Historically, spirulina has been consumed for its high nutrient value. Ancient civilizations, including the Aztecs, used it as a daily source of protein and vitamins.

5. SCIENTIFIC BENEFITS: Spirulina is exceptionally high in protein, vitamins (especially B vitamins), and essential minerals like iron and magnesium. It is rich in antioxidants, which help combat oxidative stress and may reduce inflammation. Research suggests spirulina can support cardiovascular health, boost the immune system, and may have anti-cancer properties.

6. METAPHYSICAL USES: In metaphysical practices, spirulina is used for rejuvenation and increasing energy. It is believed to enhance personal vitality and endurance and is often used in rituals aimed at health recovery and spiritual invigoration.

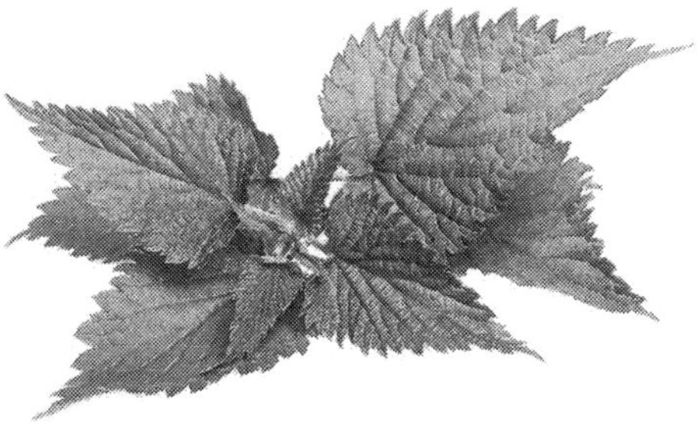

STINGING NETTLE

(URTICA DIOICA)

is a perennial flowering plant that has been used in herbal medicine since ancient times. It is well-known for its stinging hairs on the leaves and stems that inject irritants when touched.

1. DESCRIPTION: Stinging nettle plants can grow to about 2 to 4 feet tall, with opposite, heart-shaped, finely toothed leaves that are covered with tiny, hollow, stinging hairs. The plant produces small, greenish or brownish flowers.

2. LOCATION: Native to Europe, Asia, northern Africa, and western North America, stinging nettle is found in abundance in temperate climates worldwide.

3. GROWING CONDITIONS: Stinging nettle prefers rich soil with good moisture content and partial shade but can thrive in a variety of soil types. It commonly grows along riversides, in meadows, and in disturbed areas such as farm fields.

4. TRADITIONAL USES: Traditionally, nettle has been used to treat a variety of conditions, including joint pain, eczema, arthritis, gout, and anemia. It is also a popular natural remedy for urinary issues.

5. SCIENTIFIC BENEFITS: Nettle leaves are rich in nutrients, including vitamins A, C, K, and several B vitamins, as well as minerals like iron, calcium, magnesium, and potassium. It has anti-inflammatory properties and is often used to treat allergies and hay fever. The diuretic properties of nettle help with fluid retention and support kidney health.

6. METAPHYSICAL USES: In metaphysical practices, stinging nettle is used for protection and purification. It is believed to guard against negative energy, danger, and illness. Nettle is used in spells and rituals to remove curses and send back negativity sent towards someone.

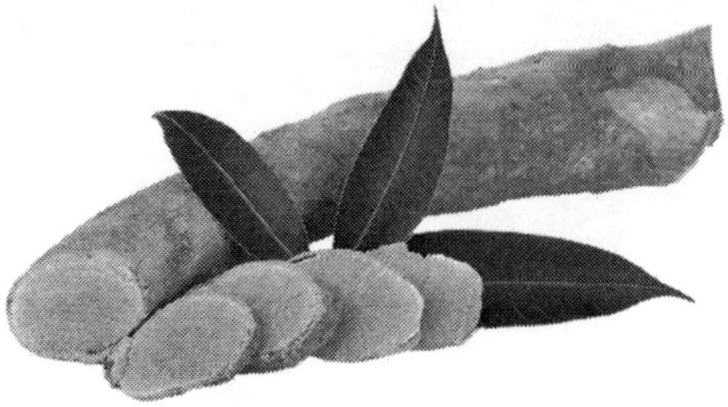

TONGKAT ALI

(EURYCOMA LONGIFOLIA)

also known as Malaysian ginseng or longjack, is a medicinal plant found in Southeast Asia. It's particularly noted for its ability to enhance male sexual health.

1. DESCRIPTION: Tongkat Ali is a tall, slender evergreen shrub-tree that can grow up to about 10 meters in height. It has compound leaves that are dark green and small, reddish or greenish-white flowers. The roots are the most commonly used part of the plant for medicinal purposes.

2. LOCATION: Native to Malaysia, Indonesia, Thailand, Vietnam, and Laos, Tongkat Ali thrives in the rainforests of Southeast Asia.

3. GROWING CONDITIONS: This plant prefers a tropical climate with plenty of rainfall. It grows well in sandy soil with good drainage and partially shaded environments but can also adapt to degraded soils.

4. TRADITIONAL USES: Traditionally, Tongkat Ali has been used to treat malaria, infections, fevers, erectile dysfunction, and as an aphrodisiac to enhance sexual performance and health.

5. SCIENTIFIC BENEFITS: The root of Tongkat Ali is rich in various compounds that may help promote male reproductive health by increasing testosterone levels, improving sperm quality, and enhancing sexual libido. It also has been studied for its potential effects on mood enhancement, as an energy booster, and for reducing stress.

6. METAPHYSICAL USES: In metaphysical practices, Tongkat Ali is often used for its energy-enhancing properties. It is believed to increase physical strength, endurance, and personal power. It is used in rituals focused on vitality, empowerment, and overcoming spiritual weakness.

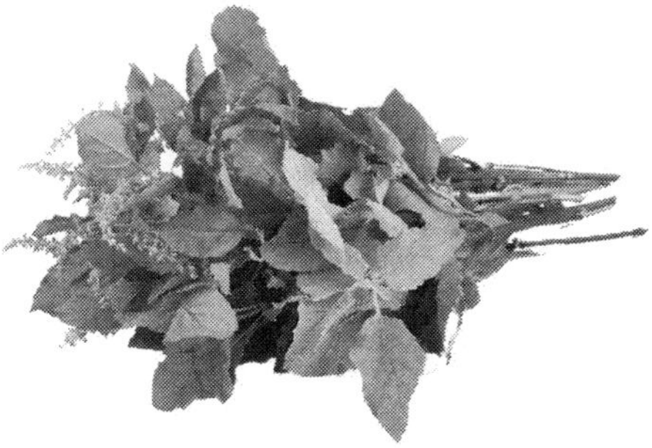

TULSI

(OCIMUM SANCTUM)

also known as Holy Basil, is a highly revered plant in Hinduism and Ayurvedic medicine. It is native to the Indian subcontinent.

1. DESCRIPTION: Tulsi is a small shrub with hairy stems, green or purple leaves, and a strong, pungent aroma. It typically grows to about 30-60 cm in height. The leaves are oval-shaped with a slightly sharp tip, and the plant produces small purple or white flowers.

2. LOCATION: While native to India, Tulsi has been cultivated throughout Southeast Asia and thrives in tropical climates.

3. GROWING CONDITIONS: Tulsi prefers full sun and rich, well-drained soil. It requires regular watering but does not tolerate overwatering or standing water.

4. TRADITIONAL USES: Tulsi is considered a sacred plant in Hindu belief and is often grown in household gardens and temples. It is traditionally used for its healing properties to treat everything from fever and diabetes to asthma and bronchitis. Tulsi is also used in teas and as an herbal remedy to reduce stress and enhance stamina.

5. SCIENTIFIC BENEFITS: Tulsi is known for its anti-inflammatory, antibacterial, and antiviral properties. It contains compounds like eugenol, which can help manage blood sugar levels, reduce cholesterol, and alleviate stress. Regular consumption of Tulsi is believed to promote longevity and enhance well-being.

6. METAPHYSICAL USES: In metaphysical practices, Tulsi is used for purification and to enhance spiritual growth. It is believed to open the heart and mind, bring clarity of thought, and promote a sense of peace. Tulsi is often used in rituals to protect and bless a home or person.

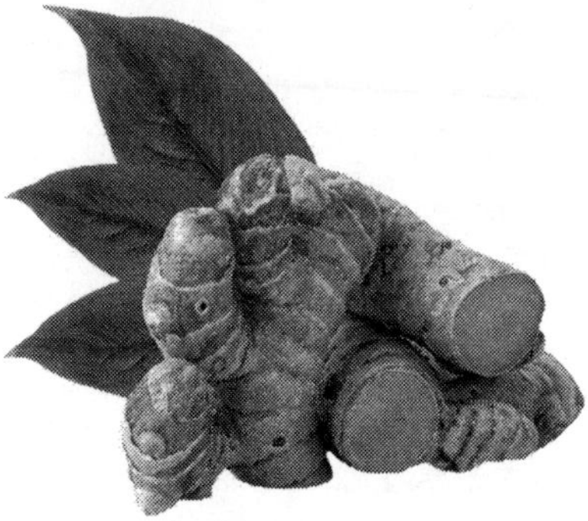

TURMERIC

(CURCUMA LONGA)

is a perennial plant of the ginger family,famous for its vibrant yellow-orange spice that comes from the root of the plant.
It is native to Southeast Asia and the Indian subcontinent.

1. DESCRIPTION: Turmeric has large, oblong leaves and a tough, brown skin with a bright orange flesh inside. It grows well in tropical climates and is cultivated primarily for its roots.

2. LOCATION: While native to India and Southeast Asia, turmeric is now widely grown in other warm and humid climates around the world, including parts of Africa and the Caribbean.

3. GROWING CONDITIONS: Turmeric thrives in temperatures between 20°C and 30°C and needs a substantial amount of annual rainfall to grow. It prefers well-drained, fertile soil and can be grown in both shaded and full sun environments.

4. TRADITIONAL USES: Traditionally, turmeric has been used in Asia for its medicinal properties, as a dye, and as a flavoring for food, especially in curry powders. It is also a vital component of Ayurvedic medicine, used to treat conditions ranging from pain and inflammation to indigestion and infections.

5. SCIENTIFIC BENEFITS: The primary active component of turmeric is curcumin, which has potent anti-inflammatory and antioxidant properties. It has been widely studied for its potential to reduce symptoms of arthritis, Alzheimer's disease, and various heart conditions. Turmeric also supports liver function and has been shown to have anticancer properties.

6. METAPHYSICAL USES: In metaphysical practices, turmeric is used for purification, protection, and healing. It is believed to cleanse the chakras, especially the solar plexus, and to help in healing by clearing negative energies. Turmeric is often used in rituals to promote energy, prosperity, and fertility.

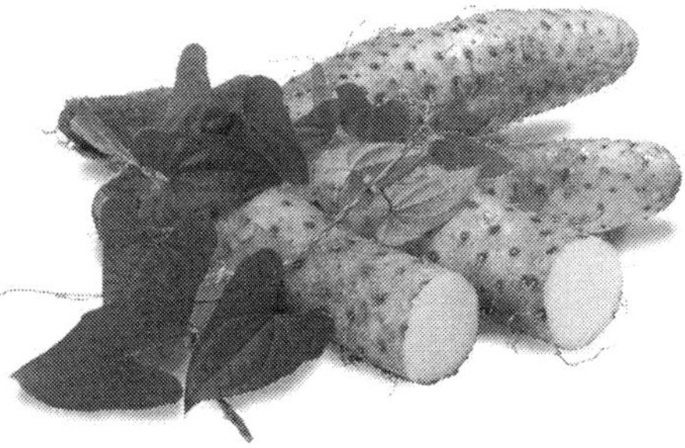

WILD YAM

(DIOSCOREA VILLOSA)

not to be confused with the yams consumed as food, is a species of a twining tuberous vine that is native to North America. It is particularly noted for its use in herbal medicine.

1. DESCRIPTION: Wild yam has heart-shaped leaves, and it produces small, inconspicuous yellowish-green flowers. The plant is most valued for its long, tuberous roots, which are rough and cylindrical.

2. LOCATION: Native to North America, wild yam grows extensively in the eastern and central United States.

3. GROWING CONDITIONS: It prefers a sunny or partially shaded habitat with moist, well-drained soil. Wild yam vines can be found climbing over rocks and other plants in wooded areas.

4. TRADITIONAL USES: Traditionally, wild yam has been used to treat a variety of ailments such as rheumatoid arthritis, menstrual cramps, digestive issues, and to ease childbirth. It was used by Native Americans to relieve colic and to soothe inflammation.

5. SCIENTIFIC BENEFITS: Wild yam contains a chemical called diosgenin, which has been used to produce steroids like estrogen and dehydroepiandrosterone (DHEA) in the laboratory. It is commonly used in alternative medicine today for its potential to relieve menopause symptoms, such as hot flashes and night sweats. Its anti-inflammatory properties also make it popular for treating arthritis.

6. METAPHYSICAL USES: In metaphysical practices, wild yam is used for grounding and balancing energy. It is believed to help soothe emotional instability and to aid in aligning the sacral and solar plexus chakras, promoting a sense of calm and balance.

HONEYS

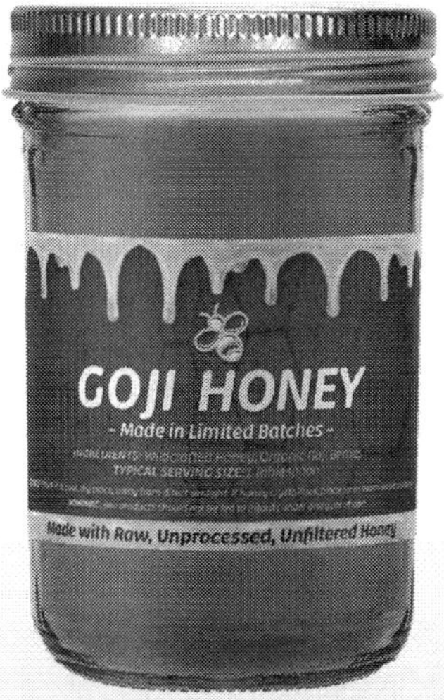

GOJI HONEY

is a unique fusion of raw honey and goji berries (Lycium barbarum), both of which are celebrated for their health benefits and distinct flavors.

1. DESCRIPTION: This infusion marries the natural sweetness and antimicrobial properties of honey with the tart, slightly sweet flavor and nutritional richness of goji berries, resulting in a reddish, nutrient-packed honey.

2. PERCEIVED BENEFITS: The combination of honey and goji berries in Goji Honey offers several health advantages:

3. ANTIOXIDANT POWER: Goji berries are loaded with antioxidants like zeaxanthin and lycopene, which help combat oxidative stress and reduce the risk of chronic diseases. When combined with the natural antioxidants found in honey, this infusion becomes a potent supporter of overall cellular health.

4. IMMUNE SUPPORT: Honey is well-known for its antibacterial and anti-inflammatory properties, which can aid in soothing infections and boosting the immune system. The addition of goji berries, which contain vitamins C and A, further enhances this benefit, making Goji Honey a strong ally during cold and flu season.

5. ENERGY AND VITALITY: Goji berries have been used historically to increase energy and vitality. Infusing these berries with honey not only enhances flavor but also provides a steady supply of natural sugars and nutrients that can help maintain energy levels throughout the day.

6. DIGESTIVE HEALTH: Honey is gentle on the stomach and can help counteract indigestion and soothe the digestive tract. Combined with the high fiber content in goji berries, Goji Honey can support digestive health and promote regularity.

7. METAPHYSICAL USES: In metaphysical practices, Goji Honey is used to promote a sense of wellness and energetic balance. It is believed to harmonize body, mind, and spirit, enhancing one's vibrational energy and providing protective qualities against negative energies.

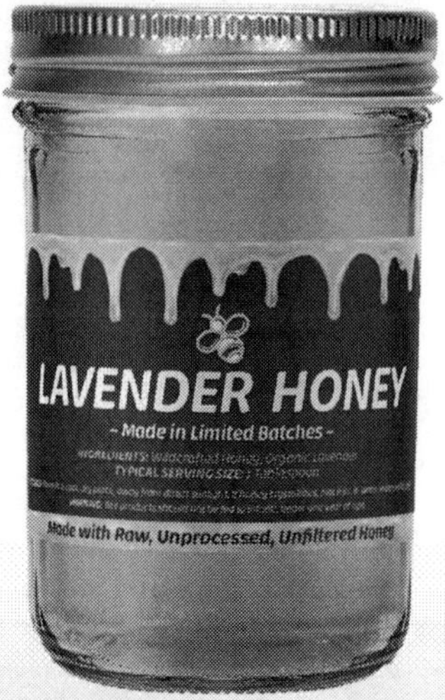

LAVENDER HONEY

is made by infusing raw honey with lavender flowers (Lavandula spp.), combining the aromatic floral notes of lavender with the sweet richness of honey.

1. DESCRIPTION: Lavender Honey features the fragrant, soothing qualities of lavender paired with the natural sweetness and beneficial properties of honey. The result is a light, fragrant honey often used in both culinary and medicinal applications.

2. PERCEIVED BENEFITS: The combination of lavender and honey in Lavender Honey offers various health advantages:

   o Relaxation and Sleep: Lavender is renowned for its calming and relaxing properties, often used to improve sleep quality and reduce anxiety. When infused with honey, which itself promotes relaxation through its antioxidants, Lavender Honey becomes a powerful aid in enhancing bedtime routines and improving overall sleep.

   o Antioxidant and Anti-inflammatory: Both lavender and honey possess antioxidant and anti-inflammatory properties. This makes Lavender Honey beneficial for reducing oxidative stress and inflammation in the body, potentially supporting skin health and speeding up healing processes.

   o Respiratory Health: Lavender has traditionally been used to treat respiratory issues. Infused in honey, it can help soothe coughs and sore throats, making Lavender Honey a comforting remedy during cold and flu season.

   o Digestive Aid: Lavender helps relieve symptoms of indigestion, stomach upset, and bloating. Combined with honey's soothing effects on the digestive tract, Lavender Honey can aid in digestion and act as a gentle remedy for digestive discomfort.

3. METAPHYSICAL USES: In metaphysical practices, Lavender Honey is often utilized for its ability to promote tranquility and emotional healing. It is used in rituals and spells aimed at bringing peace, enhancing meditation, and clearing negative energies.

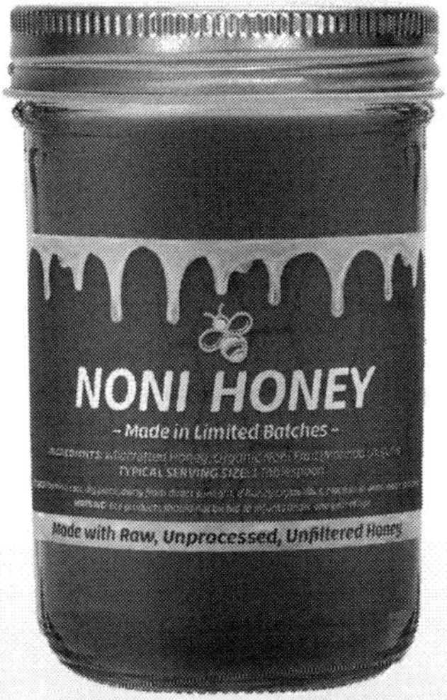

NONI HONEY

involves the infusion of raw honey with the juice or extract of the noni fruit (Morinda citrifolia), known for its distinctive flavor and a wide array of health benefits.

1. DESCRIPTION: Noni Honey combines the intense, somewhat tart flavor of noni fruit with the natural sweetness of honey. This fusion not only enhances the palatability of noni but also augments its nutritional profile.

2. PERCEIVED BENEFITS: The integration of noni with honey in Noni Honey offers several health benefits:

   o Immune System Support: Noni is rich in vitamin C and other antioxidants that help boost the immune system. When combined with the antibacterial properties of honey, Noni Honey becomes a potent dietary supplement for enhancing immune function.

   o Anti-inflammatory Properties: Both noni and honey have anti-inflammatory effects. Noni Honey can be particularly beneficial in reducing inflammation throughout the body, which is helpful for conditions like arthritis and other inflammatory diseases.

   o Energy Boost: Noni is often used as an energy booster due to its high levels of B vitamins, which are crucial for converting food into energy. Mixed with honey, which provides a quick source of natural sugar, Noni Honey can be an excellent energy enhancer.

   o Digestive Health: Noni has been traditionally used to aid digestion and soothe stomach ailments. The soothing properties of honey make Noni Honey a gentle remedy for digestive issues, promoting overall digestive health.

3. METAPHYSICAL USES: In metaphysical practices, Noni Honey is used for purification and renewal. It is believed to cleanse the body and spirit of toxins and negative energies, promoting physical and spiritual healing.

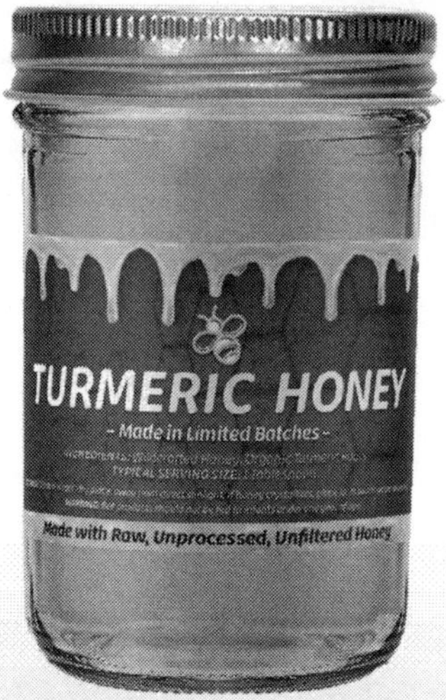

TURMERIC HONEY

is created by blending raw honey with turmeric powder (Curcuma longa), a spice renowned for its vibrant color, unique flavor, and extensive health benefits.

1. DESCRIPTION: This infusion combines the earthy, slightly bitter flavor of turmeric with the sweet richness of honey, resulting in a golden-hued honey with both culinary and medicinal appeal.

2. PERCEIVED BENEFITS: Turmeric Honey offers a range of health benefits due to the potent properties of its components:

   - Anti-inflammatory and Antioxidant Effects: Turmeric is famous for its active ingredient, curcumin, which has powerful anti-inflammatory and antioxidant properties. Mixed with honey, known for its own antioxidant abilities, Turmeric Honey is a strong supporter of overall health, helping to reduce inflammation and combat oxidative stress.
   - Immune Boosting: The antimicrobial properties of both honey and turmeric make Turmeric Honey a beneficial ally in boosting the immune system and fighting off infections.
   - Digestive Health: Turmeric promotes healthy digestion and can relieve symptoms of bloating and gas. Honey complements this by soothing the digestive tract. Together, Turmeric Honey can be a helpful dietary supplement for maintaining a healthy digestive system.
   - Skin Health: Applied topically, Turmeric Honey can enhance skin health due to turmeric's antiseptic properties and honey's hydrating effects. It's often used in masks to combat acne and brighten the skin.

3. METAPHYSICAL USES: In metaphysical practices, Turmeric Honey is used to promote healing and protection. It is believed to cleanse both physical and spiritual toxins, fostering an environment of recovery and protection from negativity.

ADDITIONAL WELLNESS TITLES

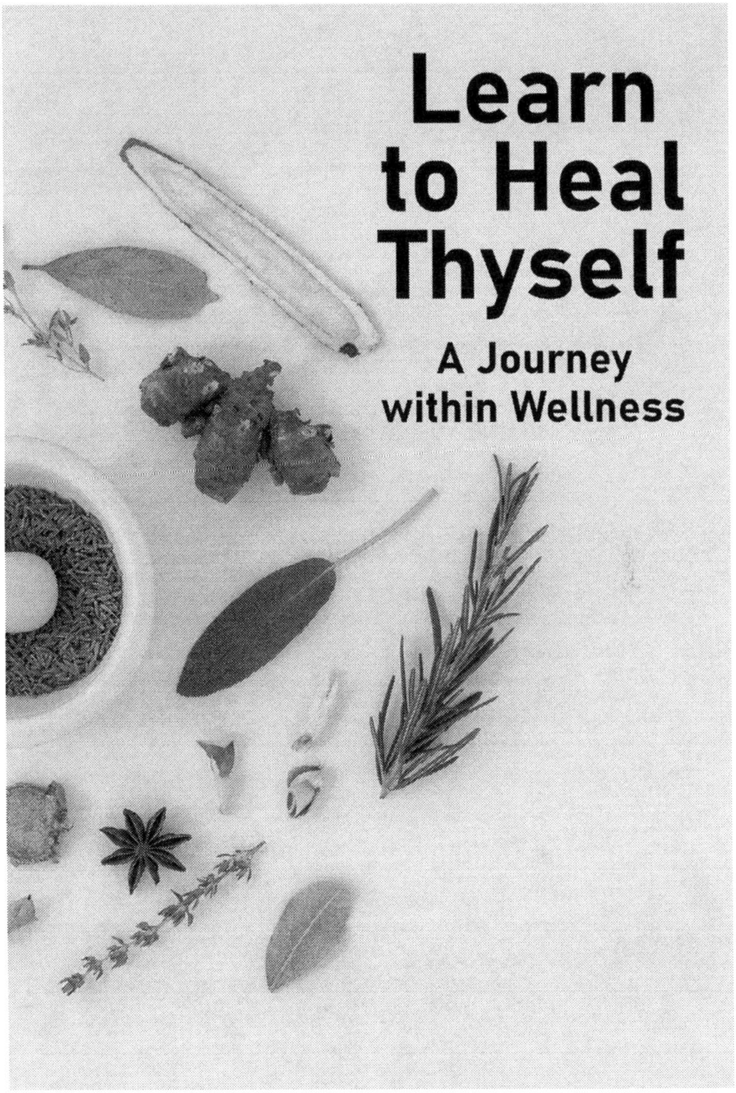
Learn
to Heal
Thyself
A Journey
within Wellness

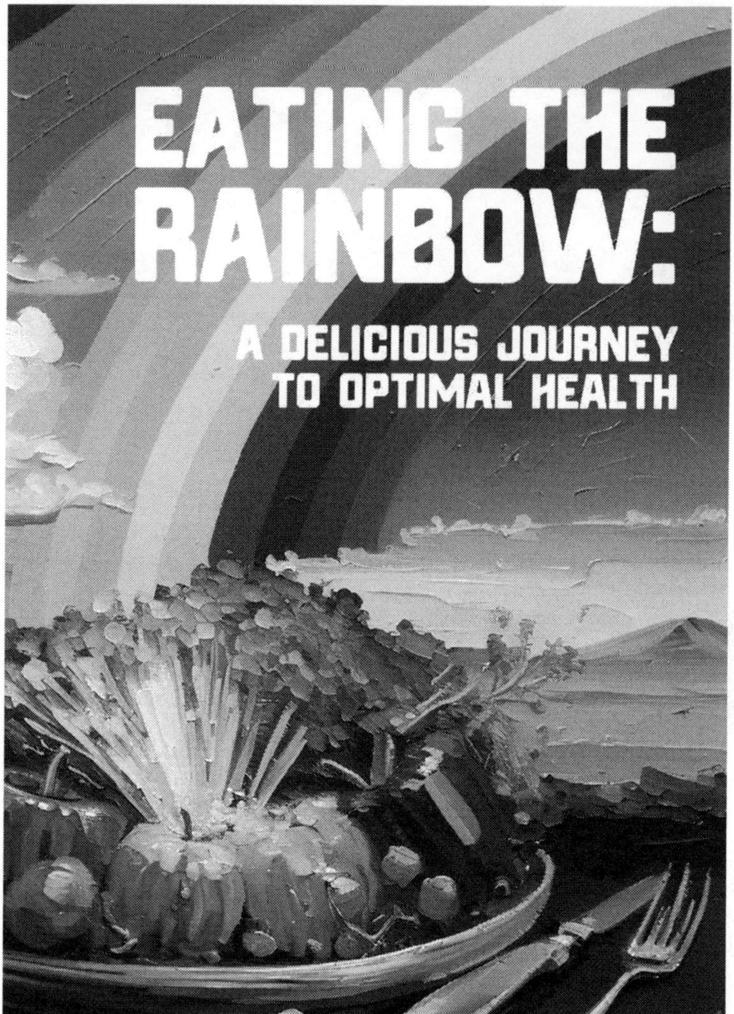
EATING THE RAINBOW:
A DELICIOUS JOURNEY TO OPTIMAL HEALTH

Made in the USA
Monee, IL
08 November 2026

67971941R00046